A GIFT OF LIFE

PROFESSOR ROY CALNE

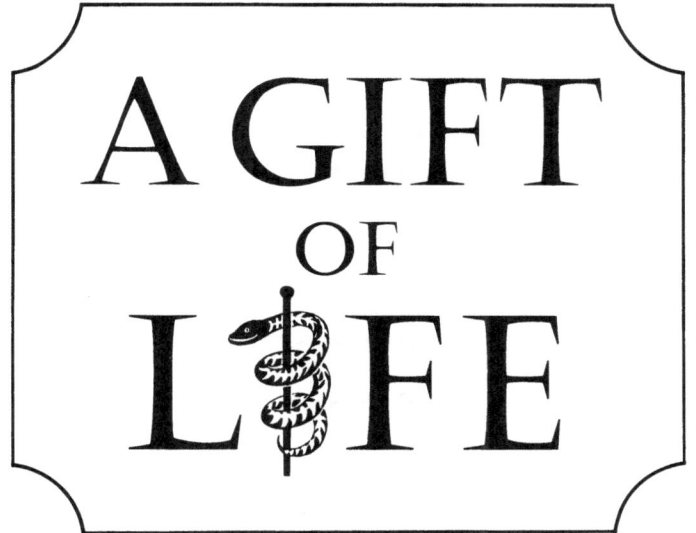

A GIFT OF LIFE

OBSERVATIONS ON
ORGAN TRANSPLANTATION

MTP

MEDICAL AND TECHNICAL
PUBLISHING CO LTD

1970

PUBLISHED BY

MTP
MEDICAL AND TECHNICAL
PUBLISHING CO LTD
Chiltern House, Oxford Road
Aylesbury, Bucks

ISBN-13: 978-94-011-5895-4   e-ISBN-13: 978-94-011-5893-0
DOI: 10.1007/978-94-011-5893-0

852 0000 49

First published 1970

Designed by Bernard Crossland

BY BURGESS AND SON (ABINGDON) LTD
ABINGDON, BERKS

TO

SIR PETER MEDAWAR

WHO KINDLED MY INTEREST
IN TRANSPLANTATION
AND HAS CONTRIBUTED
SO MUCH TO THIS SUBJECT

PREFACE

In the past few years the transplantation of organs in man has received publicity unprecedented in medical history. The first heart grafts were covered by press, radio, and television on a scale equivalent to the news of the outbreak of a major war. Unwarranted and extravagant optimism has been followed by bitter criticism. This has undermined public confidence in the medical profession and seriously impeded progress in an important endeavour aimed at reducing human suffering. This unfortunate situation has arisen from widespread ignorance amongst the public and the medical profession of the background, present achievements, and future potential of organ grafting. Short statements by experts, frequently misquoted or cut short by television interviewers, and misinformed derogatory pronouncements by prejudiced medically qualified men, with no knowledge of the field, have produced a sorry state of confusion. It is the purpose of this book to attempt to clarify organ transplantation. The principles of organ transplantation are common to all organs but I will confine most of the discussion to transplantation of four vital organs, namely the kidney, liver, heart, and lung.

ROY CALNE

Cambridge
January 1970

CONTENTS

LIST OF ILLUSTRATIONS

LIST OF ILLUSTRATIONS

LIST OF ILLUSTRATIONS

ACKNOWLEDGEMENTS

I would like to thank my secretary, Miss Patricia Hagan, for her tireless devotion in typing the manuscript and my wife for proof-reading and advice. I am grateful to the Department of Photography, Addenbrooke's Hospital, and Mrs. Marian Allen for the illustrations they provided, drawings by Yvonne Miller of Oxford Illustrations Limited, and to the publishers for their encouragement and help.

CHAPTER ONE

THE IDEA

The treatment of many progressive life-threatening diseases is surgical removal of the affected organ. An infected and inflamed appendix is removed, so is a cancerous stomach. The body can function normally without the appendix; removal of the stomach, however, can impair digestion, but this may not be a serious disability. Diseases of organs essential to life such as both kidneys, both lungs, the heart, or the liver, cannot be treated in this way since although the damaged organs can be removed, death will result unless the function is replaced. To cure disease by restoring the function of a diseased organ by a biological graft is an ancient concept. Fig. 1 (frontispiece) is a reproduction of a painting of the legend of SS. Cosmas and Damian. The saints removed the cancerous leg from a sleeping man and replaced it with a healthy leg removed from a man who had recently died. According to the legend the transplant was a complete success. There was no outcry against the saints for unethical conduct, in fact their achievement has been praised by succeeding generations and depicted in numerous medieval paintings throughout Europe. The idea of cadaveric organ transplantation is therefore well established. If the organs of a dead person can save the life and prevent suffering of another human being, this is surely a good thing. The objective of therapeutic clinical organ transplantation is to restore the function of a diseased vital organ and so return to a useful and happy life a man, woman, or child who would otherwise die. There are difficulties in

I

the fulfilment of this gift of life. The surgery must be accurate and swift, the natural tendency of the body to reject the graft must be overcome and the community must be aware of the potential benefits that organ transplantation has to offer; for at present the only suitable donors of organ grafts are human beings. The relief of human suffering by organ transplantation depends on the generosity and charity of mankind.

The idea of organ transplantation remained a miraculous legend until the middle of the present century when Dr. Joseph Murray and his colleagues in Boston successfully transplanted a kidney from a healthy individual to his identical twin, who was dying from incurable kidney disease. Identical twins arise from the same egg cell, they are biologically the same person and are therefore unable to reject each others grafts. Successful surgery cures the sick twin, provided his kidney disease does not recur in the graft. The twin grafts confirmed predictions from animal experiments, that modern vascular surgery could achieve the transfer of a living organ from one man to another so that it would function normally and restore a dying man to health. I will be chiefly concerned in this book with living, functioning grafts of which a kidney transplant is an example. There are, however, other methods of providing the body with a function that it lacks.

MECHANICAL ORGAN SUBSTITUTES

The idea of manufacturing an artificial organ goes back to the legend of Daedalus and Icarus in Greek mythology (Fig. 2). They constructed prosthetic wings to escape imprisonment on an island. According to the tale, the prosthesis of Icarus came adrift at its junction with the body because the adhesive, beeswax, melted in the sun. One of the most well-known and useful prostheses is the artificial leg which, in its modern form, is functionally far superior to a leg graft, because of the poor nerve regeneration in a living

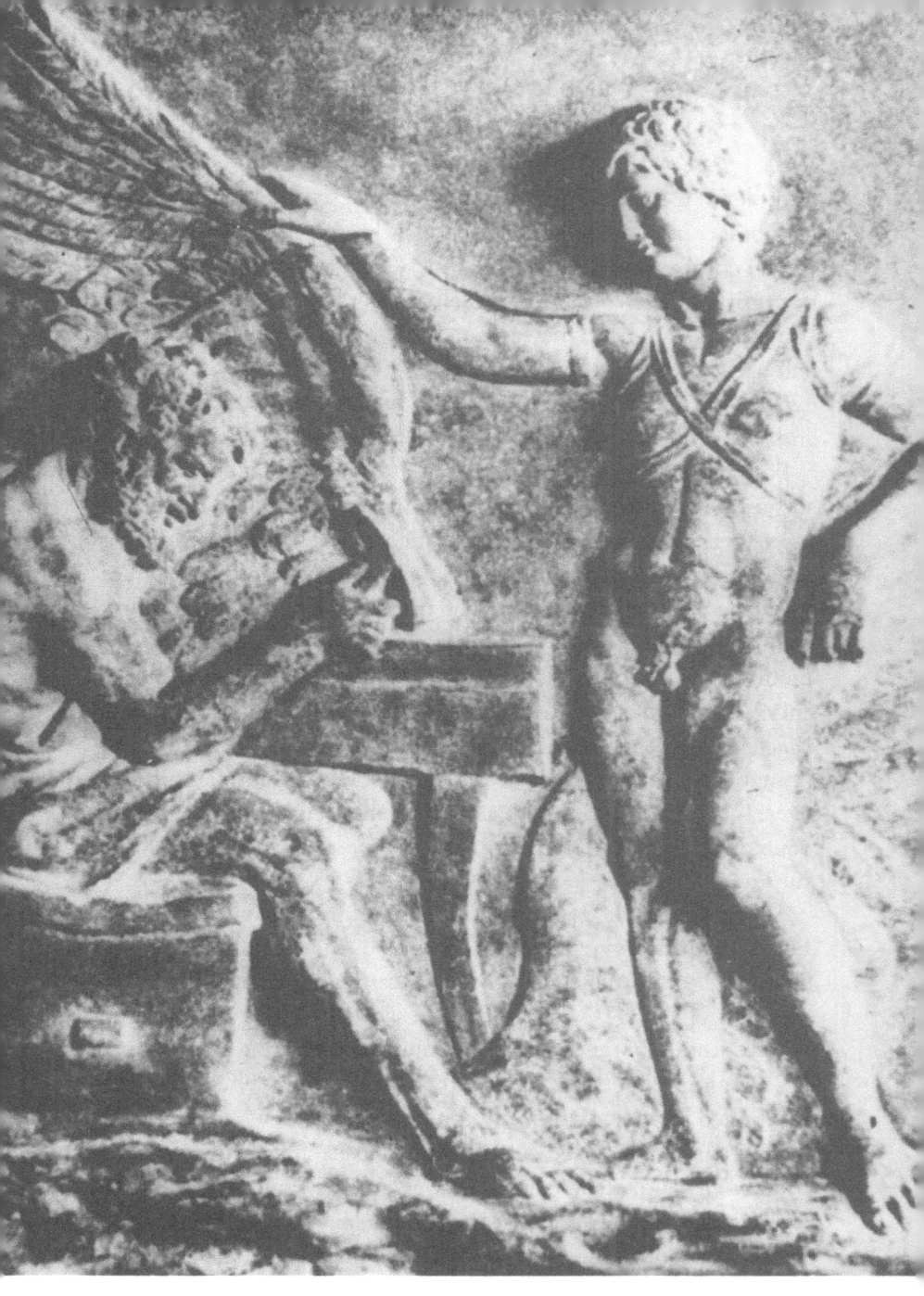

FIG. 2. Daedalus (*left*) being helped by his son Icarus in the construction of prosthetic wings. From a Roman frieze at the Villa Albani, Rome.

transplant.[1] Bone grafts provide a structural scaffold and are probably best considered as mechanical prostheses.

The cornea has rather simple functions, to protect the eye and transmit light. Corneal grafts usually fulfil these requirements, and certain inert synthetic materials may prove to be equally effective and preferable in unusual cases where grafts have failed. Countless eyes have been saved by corneal grafts, which have no blood supply and are therefore seldom rejected.

For maintenance of the circulation during and after complicated surgical procedures on the heart, the success of mechanical substitutes has been proved. Provided the mechanical heart does not have to function more than a few hours, before the patient's heart takes over, the results are excellent. The mechanical heart has pumping chambers, valves, and a supply of energy. Unfortunately no method has yet been devised of imitating the inbuilt rhythmic energy supply that is the cardinal property of normal heart muscle. Mechanical hearts are therefore cumbersome and this is the main limitation of their use as heart substitutes. Heart transplants, however, function exceedingly well provided rejection does not supervene and at present they are the only possible long-term heart substitute.

Substitutes of the lung have much in common with the heart. For short-term oxygenation of the blood, mechanical devices are excellent, but the machinery involved cannot be carried around by a patient.

Substitution of the kidney function is an interesting subject since both biological and mechanical replacements can be effective for prolonged periods. If two solutions are separated by a cellophane membrane the dissolved substances pass back and forth across the membrane until their concentrations are the same on each side. This process is called dialysis; the patient's blood containing waste products is on one side of the dialysing membrane and dialysing

1. See p. 11

4

fluid containing normal body salts is on the other. The membrane stops blood cells and protein from leaving the blood stream, but allows waste products to escape (Fig. 31). Regularly repeated haemodialysis will keep a patient in reasonable health. The disadvantages are that for fourteen hours two or three times a week the patient must be attached by his blood stream to a large, complicated, and potentially dangerous machine (Fig. 33). Moreover the points of attachment to an artery and vein of the patient have limited live sand when all have been used up dialysis is impossible. A kidney transplant is therefore preferable.

Many of the functions of the liver are unknown and since most of the vital synthetic processes of the liver that have been determined cannot be artificially reproduced, it is hardly surprising that the liver cannot be replaced by a mechanical device. For the liver, biological replacement is the only possibility.

From this brief summary of the present position of some organ substitutes, it appears that there is a continuous spectrum extending from an obvious choice of grafting for the liver, since there is no alternative, to a preference for prostheses for limbs. With other organs, replacement by either grafts or mechanical devices can be satisfactory depending on the circumstances. It is also possible to provide new parts for organs. Heart valves removed *post mortem* and manufactured valves can be grafted and will restore bedridden patients to a normal existence. Other dead grafts such as preserved arteries and bones or synthetic cloth arterial substitutes, act as functioning mechanical scaffolds into which living tissue grows. This results in their incorporation into the body as valuable prostheses.

For advances to occur in organ substitution certain difficulties must be overcome in both the mechanical and biological fields. The chief problem with mechanical organ substitution is the same as that experienced by the ill-fated Icarus, namely the junction of the prosthesis with the body. This is particularly pertinent where blood flow is required through the appliance, since blood is a complicated living tissue with a very special relationship to the physical and chemical structure of the blood vessel walls. Any roughness or changes in the electrical potential can set in motion a chain of events that result in the laying down of blood clot deposits. These may build up on the wall of the vessel and eventually occlude it or break off and block smaller vessels in the circuit. Drugs that inhibit clotting can prevent these changes but they remove the patient's defences against haemorrhage and render him vulnerable to severe bleeding from minor trauma. Also the bulk of equipment required to drive and monitor certain artificial organs is a serious impediment to the ideal solution of an implantable prosthesis. To substitute kidney function, apparatus is required that would fill the average-sized bedroom, yet a human kidney will fit into a man's hand. On the credit side, artificial organs are not attacked immunologically and this is the main, though not the only complication of biological organ grafts.

CHAPTER TWO

THE SURGERY

Every organ in the body receives its nourishment from its arterial blood supply and discharges its waste products in its venous drainage. This allows the cells of the organ to live and function. The liver has an additional blood supply which comes from the stomach and intestines, called the portal vein. The blood in this vein contains absorbed food products, minerals, and vitamins which the liver processes according to the body's needs. If the blood circulation through an organ ceases, the cells rapidly die and eventually decompose and putrify. The speed at which this occurs is governed by the temperature of the organ. Cooling slows the process. Blood circulation stops throughout the body at death, in fact cessation of circulation is the most certain criterion of death. The circulation ceases in an organ taken from a living individual as soon as the blood vessels are clamped. It follows that for a transplant to be successful, the operation must be performed quickly, whilst the cells are still capable of recovering and if the organ is cooled during the grafting operation there will be more time available in which to perform safe and accurate surgery. A minute piece of living tissue or a thin graft of skin only a few cells thick can acquire sufficient nourishment to stay alive if they are implanted into the body or laid on a surface of living cells (Fig. 3). After a few days new blood vessels grow into the graft and its early precarious existence becomes firmly established. Grafts of whole organs, however, will not survive unless their main blood vessels are immediately joined to blood

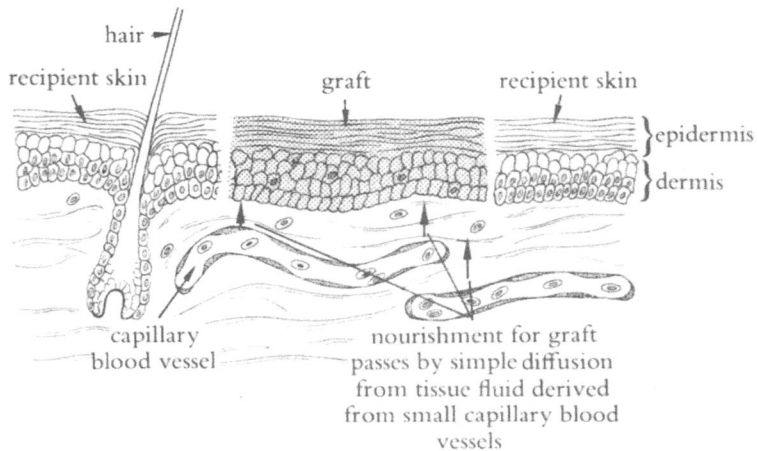

FIG. 3. Free graft of skin. Initially, it has no blood supply and gains nourishment from fluid between the cells of the recipient in the bed of the graft.

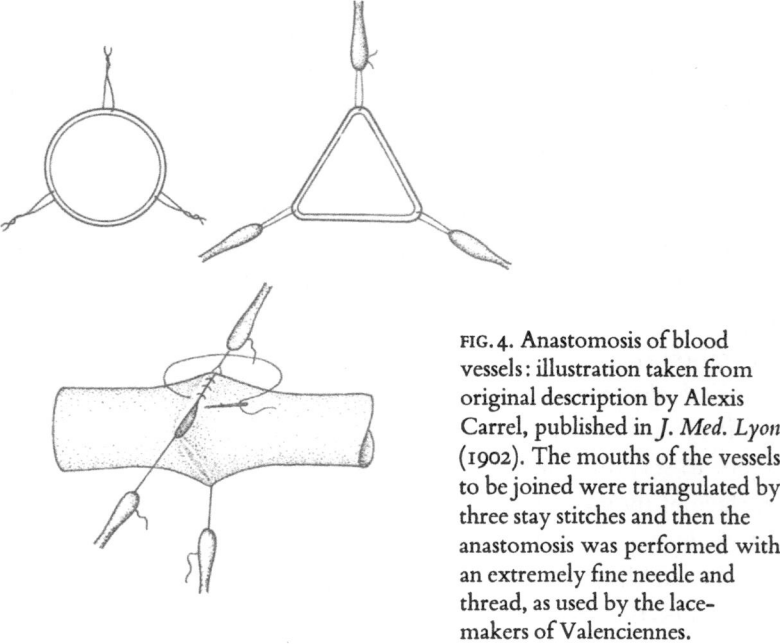

FIG. 4. Anastomosis of blood vessels: illustration taken from original description by Alexis Carrel, published in *J. Med. Lyon* (1902). The mouths of the vessels to be joined were triangulated by three stay stitches and then the anastomosis was performed with an extremely fine needle and thread, as used by the lace-makers of Valenciennes.

vessels of the recipient. Such a junction is called an anastomosis. The fate of organ grafts could not be studied until the turn of the century when Alexis Carrel described a reliable, simple method of joining blood vessels using sutures (Fig. 4). Carrel performed many of the pioneering studies on kidney transplantation in animals. He showed that kidneys transplanted by vascular anastomosis would function satisfactorily provided the time the organ was without a blood supply—the ischaemia time—was not too long. If the kidney was transplanted from its normal position to another site in the same animal (autograft) it would function indefinitely and alone support life after removal of the opposite kidney. Kidneys transplanted from one animal to another of the same species (allografts or homografts) functioned for a few days and were then rejected.

A kidney can withstand one hour at body temperature without a blood supply before permanent damage occurs. This is sufficient time in which to perform the surgery when the operation has been planned and the kidney is taken from a live donor. With human kidney transplantation from a dead donor more time is required and it is necessary to cool the organ to prevent irreversible damage (Fig. 5).

FIG. 5. Diagram of a kidney transplant. The junction of the renal artery (1) and vein (2) are shown by arrows. The ureter draining urine is implanted in the bladder (3).

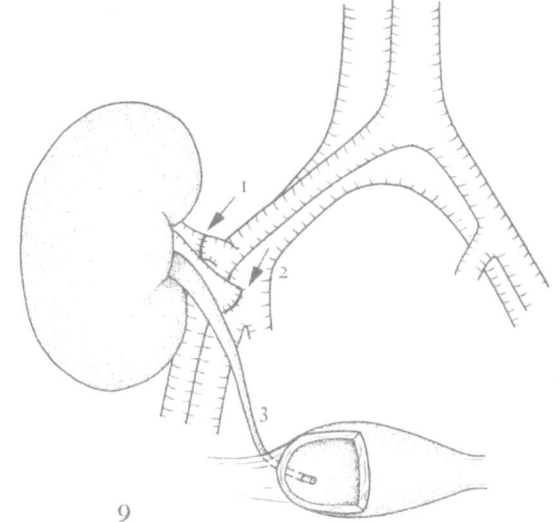

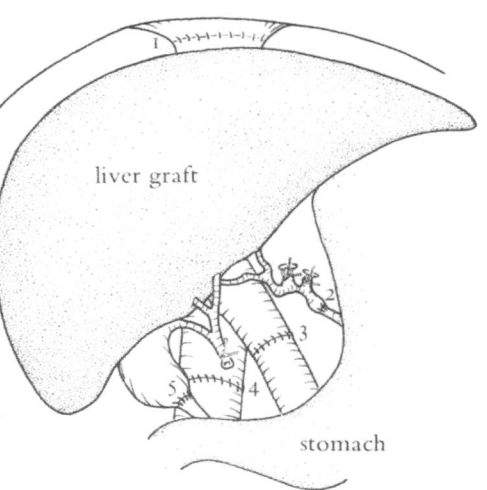

FIG. 6. Diagram of a liver transplant. The liver is placed in the correct position: orthotopic.

Anastomoses: (1) inferior vena cava above the liver, (2) hepatic artery, (3) portal vein, (4) inferior vena cava below the liver, (5) gall bladder of donor to bile duct of recipient.

liver graft

stomach

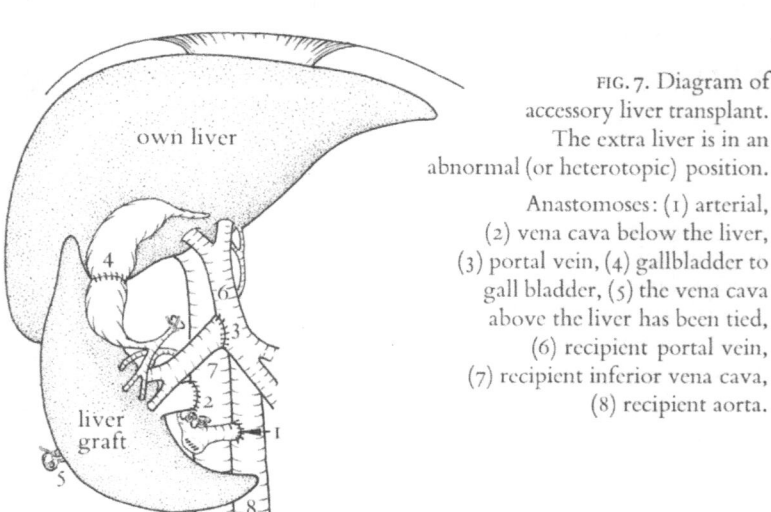

FIG. 7. Diagram of accessory liver transplant. The extra liver is in an abnormal (or heterotopic) position.

Anastomoses: (1) arterial, (2) vena cava below the liver, (3) portal vein, (4) gallbladder to gall bladder, (5) the vena cava above the liver has been tied, (6) recipient portal vein, (7) recipient inferior vena cava, (8) recipient aorta.

own liver

liver graft

An organ may be transplanted to its usual position (orthotopic) or to an abnormal site (heterotopic). Heterotopic grafts may be additional to the recipient's own corresponding organ in which case they are referred to as auxiliary or accessory grafts. Surgical details are outside the scope of this book but Figs. 6–10 illustrate some of the principles.

Surgical techniques have been developed for transplantation of all the organs of the body, including the limbs. Those illustrated, however, are likely to be the most important in clinical therapy in the foreseeable future, since failure of these organs always results in death. Replacement treatment with thyroid hormone or insulin is safer than transplantation of the thyroid or pancreas because of the attendant dangers of current anti-rejection treatment. The same argument applies to limb allografts since prostheses are preferable. One of the serious disadvantages of limb autografts—re-transplantation after accidental amputation—is that although a viable limb may result, function is likely to be impaired due to inadequate nerve regeneration. The main nerves of the limbs are mixed sensory, conveying pain, touch, temperature, and position, and motor, controlling muscle movement. No matter how carefully the nerve is joined surgically, regeneration invariably gets partly mixed with sensory nerve fibres growing into motor nerves and vice versa. In both cases the nerve will not function, resulting in impairment of both sensation and movement of the limb.

The brain or head containing the brain can be transplanted between animals, but within the brain no nerve regeneration occurs. Thus there can be no reconnection of the brain with the rest of the body. A brain transplant, although nourished with blood from the recipient, would receive no sensory information from the body, nor would it be able to control movements. Such a graft cannot be considered as a functioning transplant. Brain transplantation with all its interesting ethical and philosophical points of discussion is therefore not a serious subject. It would be a little more reasonable

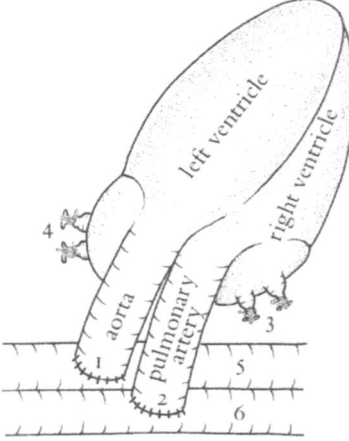

FIG.8. Heart transplant. Heart in the normal position: orthotopic.

Anastomoses: (1) right atrium, (2) left atrium, (3) aorta, (4) pulmonary artery.

FIG.9. Diagram of heart transplant in an abnormal position in the abdomen: heterotopic.

Anastomoses: (1) aorta, (2) pulmonary artery. The inferior vena cava (3) and pulmonary veins (4) have been tied, (5) recipient aorta, (6) recipient vena cava.

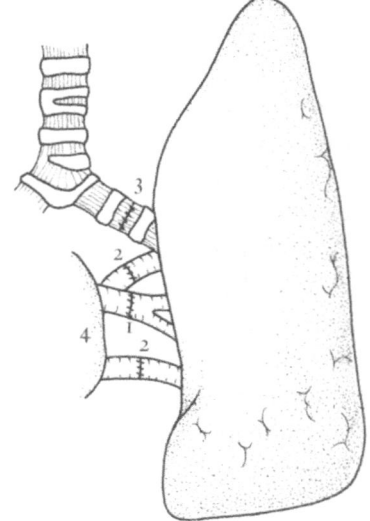

FIG. 10. Diagram of lung transplant in the correct position: orthotopic.

Anastomoses: (1) pulmonary artery, (2) pulmonary veins, (3) bronchus (airway).

to consider transplanting a new set of organs to a body shell of brain, spinal cord, peripheral nerves, and limbs. This, however, is not likely to be surgically possible in the foreseeable future and, in any case, the factors involved do not differ in principle from other organ transplantation and I will not discuss it further.

There are rare situations in which other organs might be transplanted, for example, pancreatic transplantation for insulin resistant diabetes, and intestinal transplantation for patients in whom the whole small bowel has been destroyed. If, however, rejection could be controlled readily and safely, many non-vital organs might be transplanted to the benefit of patients who at present have to suffer disability.

CHAPTER THREE

REJECTION

The tendency of the body to destroy a life-saving graft is the central point of transplantation research. Safe and predictable control of this process would be an outstanding advance, but it would be a misconception to imagine that this would, on its own, allow surgeons to transplant organs to all those in need. The serious difficulty of providing undamaged organs of suitable size in sufficient numbers would remain.

Mammalian evolution has selected in all species a powerful and complicated mechanism of defence against foreign invaders. Recovery from infection with the measles virus is accompanied by increased resistance or immunity to further invasion by this virus. The same principle operates in many infections and one of the greatest contributions of the modern era of medicine was the artificial utilization of the body's natural defence forces to produce immunity to smallpox and poliomyelitis. The importance of immunity is tragically demonstrated in rare conditions in which it is impaired. Patients unable to mount an immune response are liable to repeated and serious infections from bacteria and viruses that scarcely trouble normal people. But this life-protecting defence mechanism is unable to differentiate dangerous infective micro-organisms from life-saving grafts—hence the problem of rejection. In order to consider methods of preventing graft rejection, it is necessary to know how grafts are destroyed. Many details of this process are unknown, but I will try to summarize the established facts.

REJECTION

In the early 1940s Sir Peter Medawar and his colleagues studied the behaviour of rabbits towards skin allografts. For the first 4–5 days after grafting, allografts and autografts appeared identical, then over the next 3–4 days the allografts turned purple and gradually died, leaving a scab, whilst autografts persisted in a healthy state. If the animal was now skin grafted again from the same donor, the second graft was always destroyed more quickly than the first, whilst a graft from a third animal was rejected in the same period as the first graft. Experience of the first graft leading to its rejection had sensitized or immunized the rabbit specifically against the donor, so that a 'second-set' graft was rejected more rapidly. This pattern of reaction has been observed in all mammalian species and even in goldfish following scale grafting! It also applies to other tissues and organs. Moreover, rejection of a skin graft will immunize an animal against other tissue grafts from the same donor, for example, a kidney transplant. Thus after rejecting a skin graft at 8–10 days, a dog may destroy a kidney transplant from the same donor in 1–2 days. Following intensive research from scientists in many disciplines over the past twenty years, an incomplete though coherent picture of the rejection process has emerged. Genetic mouse-breeding experiments have shown that the factors determining the rejection or acceptance of tissue grafts are inherited and segregate in a similar manner to red blood cell groups. Breeding mice by brother/sister matings over fifteen or more generations can result in a line of inbred mice, in which the individuals have identical tissue groups called histocompatibility factors. Grafts between such mice are accepted indefinitely as though they were autografts. The principles determined in these mouse-breeding experiments have been applied to man in the search for relatively compatible donor/recipient combinations. The techniques involved in such tissue typing will be considered later.

The chemical nature of the 'histocompatibility factors' has not been fully determined. We do not yet know the subtle chemical variations that exist in the human population which can be recognized so easily and dealt with so ruthlessly by the body's immune defences. Dr. D. A. L. Davies has carefully examined different parts of body cells and has shown that the histocompatibility factors are present in the membrane that encloses the cell. A mouse injected with cell membrane from another mouse reacts against the membrane by becoming immune, so that a skin graft from the membrane donor is destroyed more rapidly than would otherwise have been expected. A substance that produces this type of specific immunity is

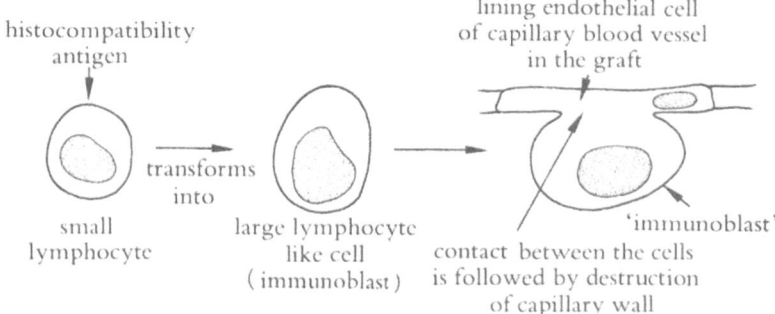

FIG. 11. Diagram of transformation of a small lymphocyte into a large lymphoid cell, immunoblast, resulting from stimulation by the histocompatibility antigens of a foreign graft. On the right the immunoblast has adhered to a capillary wall cell.

called an antigen. Cell membrane histocompatibility factors are, therefore, transplantation antigens. The membrane fractions belong to a chemical family called glycoproteins and it can be anticipated that further information on their exact composition will be obtained as research continues. The recognition of a foreign graft and its destruction is brought about by certain white blood cells called lymphocytes which are also to be found in lymph nodes, tonsils, spleen, bone marrow, and other lymphoid tissues. Forty-eight hours after a kidney allograft, small lymphocytes throughout

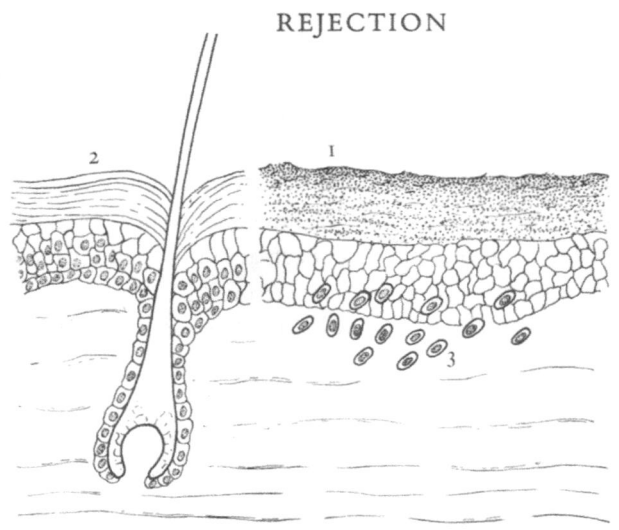

FIG. 12. Diagram of skin allograft undergoing rejection (1). The normal skin is shown adjacent to the graft (2). In the graft most of the skin cells have died as a result of immune reaction, the main signs of which are infiltration of the bed of the graft with lymphoid cells (3).

the body transform into large cells called immunoblasts which infiltrate the graft and appear to be associated with its destruction (Fig. 11). Other lymphoid cells probably change into plasma cells which produce protein antibodies which damage the graft further and may remain in the blood to destroy almost instantaneously a second graft from the same donor (or a donor with some of the same histocompatibility factors). An antibody is, therefore, a substance produced by the body in response to an antigen which reacts with and may destroy the antigen. Figs. 12–14 show the rejection process of allografted skin, heart, and kidney in the pig which usually occurs within a week of grafting.

The way in which foreign tissue is recognized and lymphoid cells are recruited is not known. The mechanism of graft destruction is also not understood, but the earliest change that can be seen in a graft is close apposition of immunoblasts to the cells that line the

REJECTION

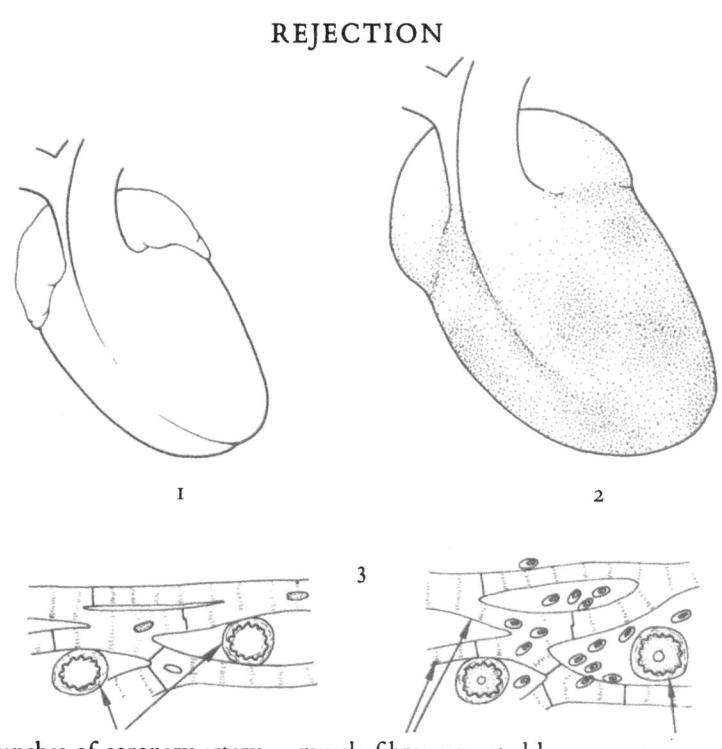

branches of coronary artery
amongst heart muscles

muscle fibres separated by
infiltrating immunoblasts

narrowed
artery

FIG. 13. Diagram showing the features of a normal heart (1) compared with a rejected heart (2). The gross appearance of the rejected heart is of enlargement, fluid accumulation (oedema), and haemorrhage. Microscopically below (3) the heart muscle fibres are shown infiltrated with lymphoid cells and the branches of the coronary artery are narrowed internally by the rejection process.

small blood vessels of the transplant. At forty-eight hours this process starts to occur and the cell membranes of both the immunoblast and cells that line the blood vessels break down where they are in contact (Fig. 15). Shortly after, the blood vessel wall disrupts, and this results in death of the tissue supplied by the blood vessel (Fig. 16). It seems likely that circulating antibodies in the blood stream can also damage the lining of the blood vessels of the graft and by narrowing their calibre impair the transplant's function (Fig. 17).

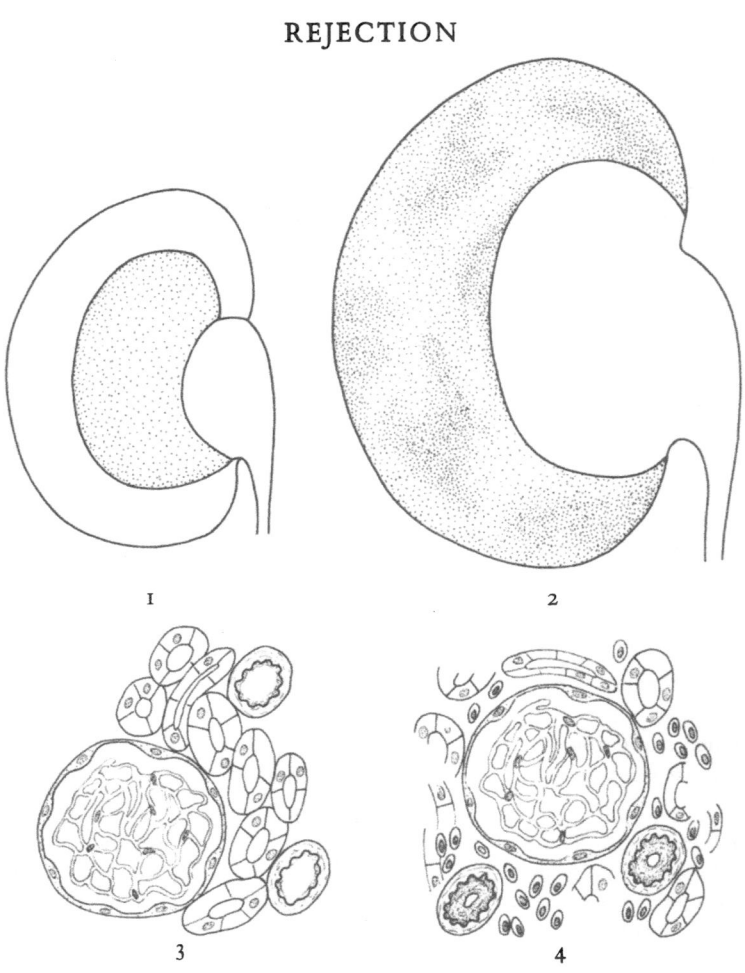

FIG. 14. Diagram of normal kidney (1), rejected kidney (2). The rejected kidney is grossly swollen with areas of oedema and haemorrhage. The microscopical changes of rejection are intense infiltration of the kidney tissue with lymphoid cells (3) and narrowing of the blood vessels (4).

From the above discussion it is apparent that although the discrete chemical interactions of tissue rejection have yet to be determined, the main features are at least partially understood and the extent of our ignorance is not sufficient to despair of a solution.

REJECTION

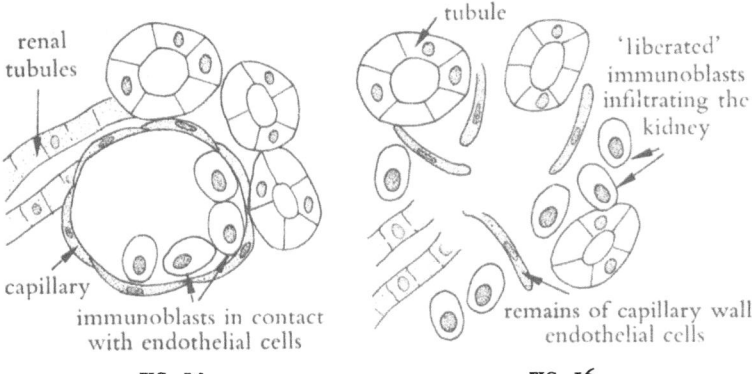

renal tubules

capillary

immunoblasts in contact with endothelial cells

FIG. 15

tubule

'liberated' immunoblasts infiltrating the kidney

remains of capillary wall endothelial cells

FIG. 16

FIG. 15. Diagram of large lymphoid cells, immunoblasts, in close contact with the endothelial cells of the capillary wall in a kidney undergoing rejection.

FIG. 16. The rejection process, more advanced than Fig. 15. The capillary wall has been broken down and the immunoblasts have been liberated into the substance of the kidney.

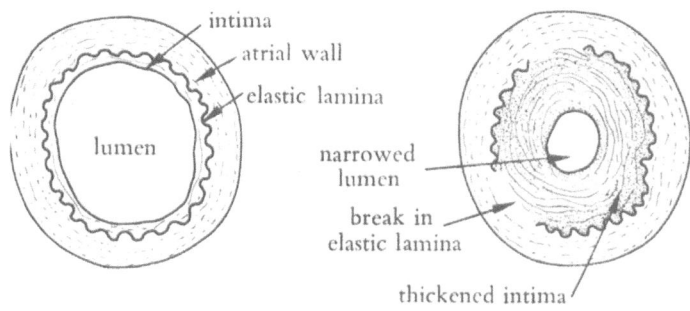

intima

atrial wall

elastic lamina

lumen

narrowed lumen

break in elastic lamina

thickened intima

FIG. 17. Diagram of the typical signs of rejection in an artery of an organ graft compared with a normal artery (*left*). After undergoing rejection (*right*) there is severe narrowing of the internal lumen which will eventually become completely blocked. The narrowing is probably the result of antibodies damaging the lining of the artery. Attempts at repair of repetitive damage result in accumulation of scar tissue which eventually blocks the vessel.

REJECTION

Diabetes is still imperfectly understood, yet control of the disease with insulin has been one of the most successful examples of effective medical treatment. By analogy the possibilities of preventing graft rejection without a full understanding of the process is not totally unreasonable.

CHAPTER FOUR

PREVENTION OF REJECTION

In the previous chapter on the rejection process, it was stated that the recipient's cells of the lymphoid family were involved in both the recognition and destruction of the grafted tissue. The evidence for this is overwhelmingly strong and it is, therefore, essential to consider the lymphoid system in any approach to the prevention of rejection.

One of the organs rich in lymphocytes which plays a central role in the development of the rest of the lymphatic tissues is the thymus. This rather insignificant gland, which lies at the base of the heart, is relatively more prominent in the embryo and young child than in adults. Lymphocytes are normally arranged in clusters called follicles, which are to be found in lymph glands throughout the body. The main activity of the thymus probably occurs during embryonic and neonatal development since its removal from new-born mice permanently impairs development of the lymphoid follicles. Functionally important areas in lymphoid follicles are dependent on the thymus for their cell population. Dr. J. A. F. P. Miller found that mice whose thymuses had been removed at birth were unable to reject skin allografts and became extremely sensitive to infections, from which they usually succumbed at an early age. The developmental phase of the lymphoid system is of great importance to the welfare of the individual, since during this phase an immune response cannot be mounted against any antigens. Sir McFarlane Burnet suggested that this phase of unresponsiveness permanently prevented the occurrence of immunity to potential antigens present during development, namely the proteins and other constituents of the individual in question. Thus during development the lymphoid system is instructed to disregard the individual's own tissues as antigens and accept them as 'self' constituents. This theory explained the normal lack of immune reaction of an individual against himself. Moreover, a defect in the process could result in the so-called auto-immune diseases; illnesses in which immune damage against the patient's own tissues does occur. This theoretical consideration remained of academic interest until further extremely important experiments were performed by Sir Peter Medawar and his colleagues in the 1950s. An investigation of skin grafts between non-identical cattle twins led to the unexpected result that the grafts were accepted indefinitely as though the animals had been identical twins. Now it was known that a peculiarity of non-identical cattle twins is a mixing of blood between the embryos *in utero* and the coexistence of red cells of different blood groups in the individual calves which persisted into adult life. These observations fitted Burnet's hypothesis very neatly. Thus it was argued that the exchange of blood between the embryo calves presented the developing lymphoid systems with both red cell and white cell antigens of the other twin. Since the white blood cells contain histocompatibility antigens, the calves would treat their respective twin's antigens as their own and be unable to react against them when, at a later stage, skin was grafted from their twin. The non-identical twin calves tolerated each other's tissues and the phenomenon was called 'natural immunological tolerance'. Proof that this reasoning was correct was provided by deliberate injection of embryonic neonatal mice with tissue from an unrelated mouse. Later the injected animals were challenged with grafts from the same donor source which provided the injection.

PREVENTION OF REJECTION

Such grafts were accepted, whilst grafts from third party animals as distinct from the original donor and recipient, were rejected normally. This experimentally induced 'immunological tolerance' was therefore specific for the donor in question and did not produce generalized impairment of the defence mechanisms. A further interesting finding was a wasting disease which developed in mice made tolerant by the injection of lymphoid cells from adult donor mice. This was an immunological illness called 'runt' disease, in which the recipient was powerless to destroy the injected cells, but the

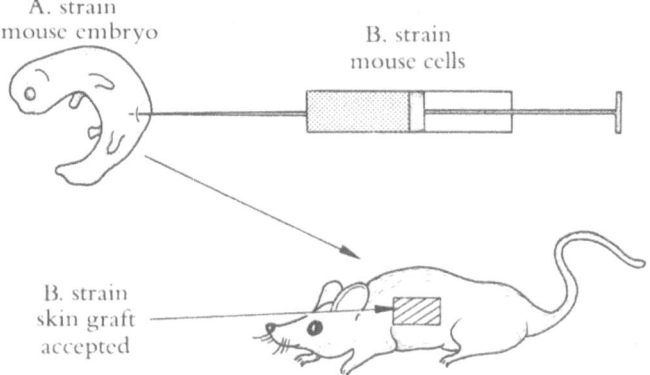

If adult immunologically competent lymphoid cells are injected into the embryo, it may become a 'runt' due to an immune reaction of the grafted lymphoid cells against the host

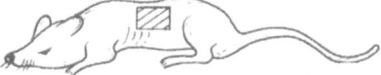

FIG. 18. Diagram of the experimental induction of immunological tolerance. The A strain mouse embryo has an immature lymphoid system which cannot react against the injected B strain cells and accepts them as though they were its own. Thus subsequent B strain skin grafts are permanently accepted. If the injected cells are adult lymphocytes they can react against A strain histocompatibility antigens and produce a wasting graft versus host reaction called 'runt' disease.

injected cells being lymphocytes were able to mount an immune attack against the histocompatibility antigens of the injected mouse. This was a 'graft versus host reaction' and had similarities to some autoimmune diseases in man (Fig. 18).

The goal of transplantation research is to provide permanent acceptance of the grafted organ with no other unpleasant side-effects. Immunological tolerance was the first demonstration that such graft acceptance could be achieved between unrelated individuals, but the necessity for the toleragenic injection to be given during development prevented classical tolerance from being utilized in clinical treatment. The mechanism by which tolerance is produced has been extensively investigated, but how antigen can confer such a profound, specific, and long-lasting effect on the lymphoid system is still not known. It has been shown, however, that in the first few days after birth it becomes increasingly difficult to render mice tolerant. A larger dosage of cells must be injected and the state of tolerance becomes less complete, so that skin grafts from the donor source may be slowly rejected after prolonged acceptance. Eventually even massive cell dosage can no longer produce tolerance. Studies on the induction of tolerance to simple protein antigens, for instance human albumin injected into mice, have shown that the route of injection and the dose can be critical. Antigen injected directly into the blood stream is more likely to produce tolerance than when it is injected into or under the skin. Tolerance to simple proteins may be induced by minute doses, larger amounts will produce the opposite of tolerance, namely immunity, whilst huge doses may again produce tolerance. With transplantation antigens, the closer the relationship of donor to recipient the easier it is to produce tolerance. I feel that it is necessary to understand these rather complicated features of tolerance in order to appreciate the discussion which follows.

When a graft is maintained without rejection by the currently popular immunosuppressive drugs, it has frequently been shown that after some months the drug dosage may be reduced, and rarely even stopped, without the graft being rejected and with the obvious advantage to the patient that he becomes less liable to develop serious infections. This adaptation is probably specific and results

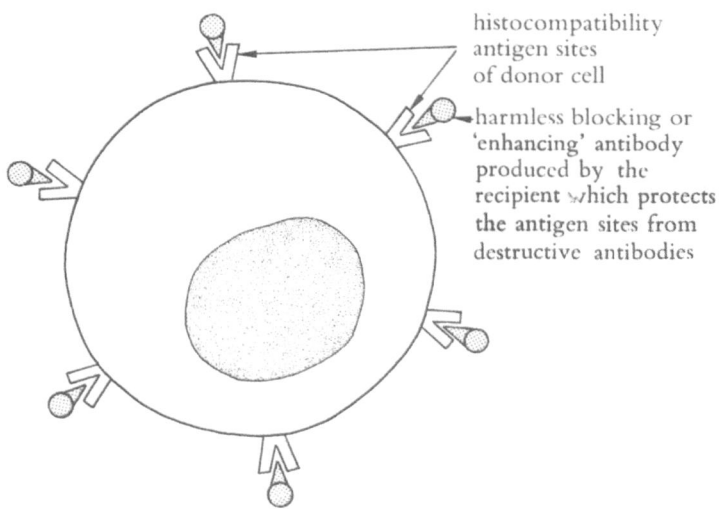

histocompatibility antigen sites of donor cell

harmless blocking or 'enhancing' antibody produced by the recipient which protects the antigen sites from destructive antibodies

FIG. 19. Diagram to show a possible explanation of one of the methods of prolonged graft acceptance. Specific non-toxic antibodies produced by the recipient render the donor cell non-antigenic because they block the antigen sites.

from changes both in the graft and the host. It seems likely that the changes in the host involve a partial state of tolerance, whilst the graft changes appear to be the result of a specific deletion of relevant antigenic histocompatibility factors in the graft. How this latter change is brought about is not definitely known, but experimental observations suggest that it is due to a specific blocking or 'enhancing' antibody produced by the host, which does not destroy the grafted cells, but covers up their antigenic sites so that they no longer act as antigens (Fig. 19).

Although many attempts have been made to induce tolerance to allografts in animals with mature immune defences there was little success until some unexpected results occurred in grafting experiments in the pig. Skin, kidney, and heart allografts are rejected by the pig, usually within one week, the features of rejection being the same as those in other species (Figs. 12–14). Liver grafts in the pig, however, often survive indefinitely. Small three-month-old pigs, quite capable of mounting an immune response, will thrive following liver grafting. The transplant grows with the pig and animals have gained an eightfold weight increase. One sow delivered a litter of nine normal piglets eighteen months after liver allografting and removal of her own liver (Fig. 20). This remarkable difference of behaviour towards liver grafts compared with other tissues was investigated further by grafting other tissues from the same or different donors to the recipient at the time of liver grafting. The liver conferred protection from rejection on grafts of skin, heart, and kidney from the liver donor. Similar grafts from other indifferent donors were usually rejected at the normal time, occasionally they also had prolonged survival, but never as long as the grafts from the liver donor.

FIG. 20. Nine piglets suckling from their mother, whose own liver was removed and replaced with an orthotopic liver graft eighteen months previously. The animal was given no immunosuppressive treatment. (By courtesy of *Nature*)

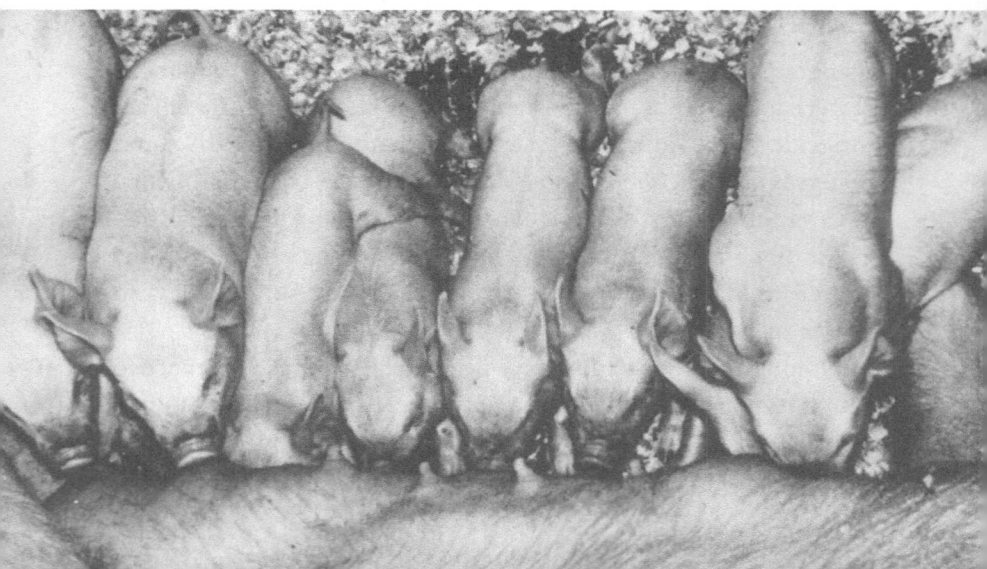

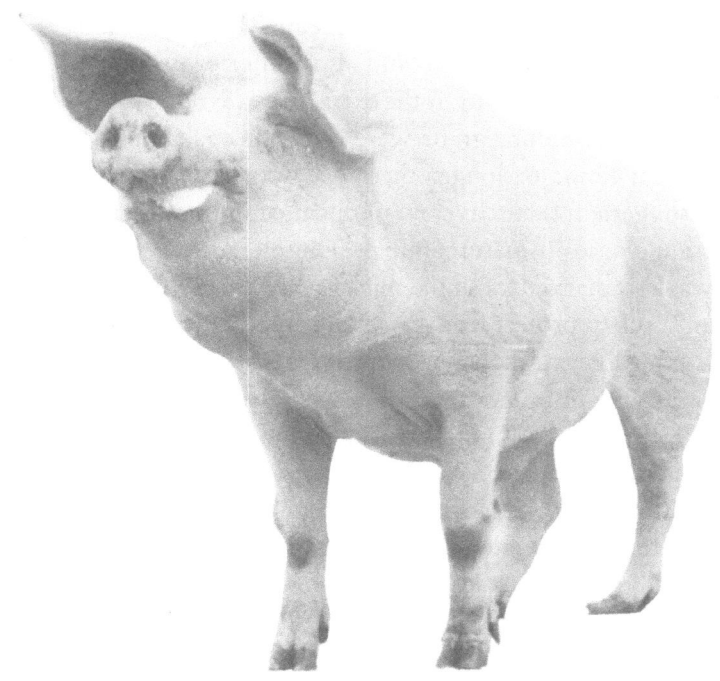

FIG. 21. A pig that had both its own kidneys and liver removed. It received a liver and kidney graft from the same donor and was given no immunosuppressive treatment. More than two years later the animal has developed normally and is very well.

The specific protective effect was greatest for the liver itself but also profound for the kidney. Skin grafts survived two to three times longer than normal and following their rejection the liver continued functioning normally and was not rejected. A few experiments on the heart suggested that it was protected for longer than skin and shorter than the kidney. Fig. 21 shows a healthy pig more than two years after liver and kidney grafting from the same donor and removal of its own liver and both kidneys. Note though, that pigs sensitized first by kidney grafts are capable of rejecting a subsequent liver graft rapidly. The protective effect of a liver graft does not depend on removal of the recipient's liver since accessory livers are not usually rejected and also confer protection on other donor specific tissue grafts. If the extra liver was removed after two hours, skin and kidney grafts were not protected, but if it was left twentyfour hours or longer there was protection. These experiments suggested that the liver was inducing immunological tolerance in immunologically mature animals. The tolerance was not complete and was least marked for skin, which has always been the most recalcitrant tissue to protect from rejection. In other species skin, heart, kidney, and liver are in that order progressively easier to maintain as allografts with immunosuppressive drugs. It seems possible that the liver grafts in the pig induce partial immunological tolerance by releasing suitable amounts of histocompatibility antigen in a chemical form that overrides the immunity-producing tendency of antigens that are liberated from skin, heart, or kidney grafts.

It will be of interest to test this hypothesis by attempting to reproduce the protective effects of a liver graft with antigenic extracts of liver. The results of the porcine experiments described above could be unique to the pig, but it is likely that they are of more general biological relevance, the pig being a species in which the phenomenon can be most easily demonstrated. Fig. 22 shows a Rhesus monkey given no immunosuppressive treatment which did not reject a liver allograft after seven months, yet this species usually rejects skin, kidney, and heart allografts after a week.

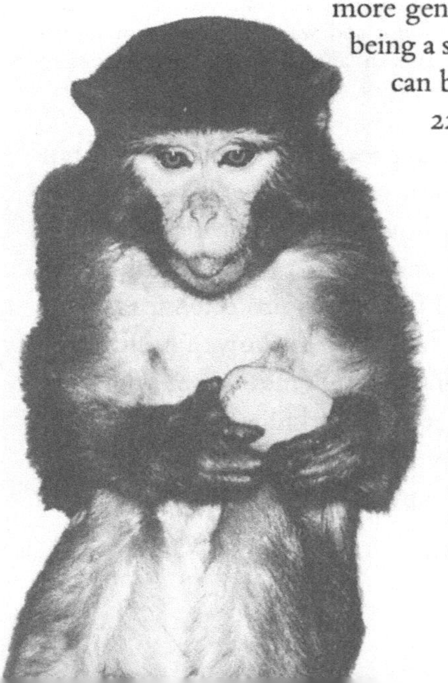

FIG. 22. A Rhesus monkey which had its own liver removed and received an orthotopic liver graft from another Rhesus monkey. The animal was given no immunosuppressive drugs and lived for seven months after operation. It died from an infection.

PREVENTION OF REJECTION

The discussion of specific antigen-induced protection of grafts from rejection or tolerance has been deliberately rather detailed, since this is our eventual aim in human organ transplantation. Less satisfactory immunosuppressive measures are available and will now be considered. They all act by removing, destroying, or damaging the lymphoid cell population and as a consequence when effective they impair the body's defence against infection. Numerous immunosuppressive agents and regimens have been described, but most of these are inferior in activity and additive in toxicity to the three main agents Imuran, adrenal steroids, and anti-lymphocyte serum. Destruction of lymphocytes with X-irradiation was the first method of immunosuppression to be extensively studied. Unfortunately the dose of X-rays required to prevent allograft rejection destroyed the bone marrow and damaged the intestines. In order to prevent the irradiated animals from dying it was necessary to give them bone marrow grafts. Since the X-rays had destroyed the immune system, there was a serious danger that the injected bone marrow cells would mount an immune attack on the recipient and produce a graft v. host secondary wasting disease, similar to 'runt' disease which could be lethal. In spite of these hazards some animals survived the X-rays and marrow grafting and would then accept skin grafts from the bone marrow donors without protest. Application of total body irradiation to kidney transplantation in man was usually unsuccessful. Sufficient X-ray dosage to prevent rejection killed the patient, whilst less drastic dosage resulted in inability to prevent rejection of the kidney allograft. Attempts to obtain selectivity with irradiation have not been conspicuously encouraging. Two approaches have been tried. Firstly to irradiate the grafted organ. This destroys lymphocytes infiltrating the graft, but may also damage the transplant. Secondly to irradiate the patient's blood or lymph outside the body to destroy circulating lymphoid cells and then return the lymphocyte-depleted blood or lymph to the circulation. Modifications of this approach used experimentally have been to implant an irradiating source in a large blood vessel within the animal, or to inject radio-active material into the lymphatic system to destroy the lymph nodes. It is doubtful whether these techniques will be of significant therapeutic value. Removal of lymphocytes by external drainage of the main lymphatic vessel, the thoracic duct, certainly depletes the lymphocyte population rapidly and was shown by Professor Gowans to increase skin graft survival two to three times longer than normal. It has not, however, yet been clearly shown that the effects add significantly to the immunosuppression used routinely in clinical organ transplantation.

Imuran (azathioprine)

This drug is closely related to 6-mercaptopurine (6-MP) which is a very useful anti-leukaemic agent. In 1959 6-MP was found to impair the ability of rabbits to produce antibodies against injected foreign proteins. Kidney allografts in dogs were also protected from rejection by this drug (Fig. 23). A search was made for a similar chemical which might have less toxic side-effects than 6-MP and its derivative Imuran was found to be slightly preferable. It can be given by mouth, but the dosage has to be carefully moni-tored since it may damage the bone marrow and lead to disastrous infections and haemorrhage. People vary greatly in their suscepti-bility to Imuran and initially the white blood cell and platelet counts must be determined daily to avoid overdosage. Neverthe-less Imuran is an extremely valuable drug and has been used as the sheet anchor of immunosuppressive treatment in most patients with organ grafts. High doses are given initially, but after three to four months, if the transplant is functioning well, the dose is cautiously diminished, but most patients do require con-tinuation of treatment indefinitely. Even minute doses, years after transplantation, may be essential to maintain a peaceful coexistence

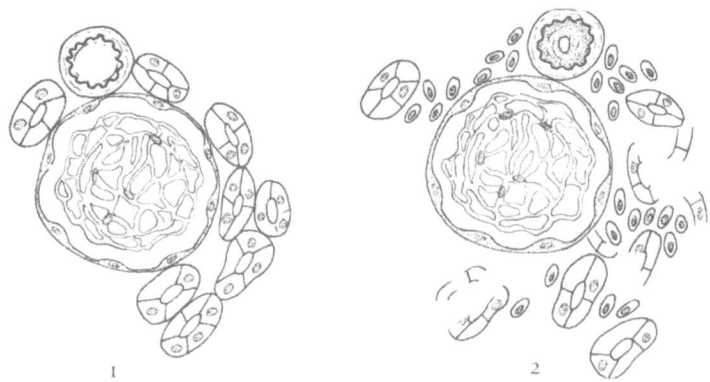

FIG. 23. Diagram of a kidney allograft at *six months* in an animal treated with azathioprine (1) compared with a similar kidney allograft at *seven days* in an animal receiving no immunosuppressive treatment (2). There is no evidence of rejection at six months in the treated animal compared with very severe cell infiltration, arterial damage, and death of kidney cells in the untreated animal.

between graft and host. The exact mode of action of Imuran is unknown; it belongs to a category of drugs called antimetabolites and its chemical structure is similar to that of the essential purine base, adenine, which is a constituent of nucleic acids and certain important enzyme systems. Antimetabolites are believed to act by competing with the natural substances to which they are chemically related, but having perpetrated this chemical fraud, the antimetabolite cannot fulfil the biological function of the natural metabolite and the result is malfunction or death of the affected cells. Imuran certainly kills fast-dividing cells such as those of the bone marrow and intestines, but it has a selective action in inhibiting the immune response against grafted organs at relatively nontoxic dosage and this makes it useful in practice.

Adrenal cortical steroids

In view of their powerful anti-inflammatory and lymphocyte depletion actions, it not surprising that Cortisone and its close relatives Prednisone and Prednisolone, are also useful in prolonging allograft survival. Like Imuran, Prednisone or Prednisolone can be given by mouth. They are not toxic to the bone marrow, but they predispose the body to infections and slow wound healing. Large doses have many unpleasant side-effects and can produce all the features of adrenal cortex overactivity called 'Cushing's Syndrome'. The patients develop a bloated complexion and their faces swell. They tend to gain weight, become diabetic, and the bones may be demineralized. Efforts are therefore made to avoid prolonged high dosage with steroids, but unfortunately few patients can be maintained without these drugs, which are particularly valuable during acute rejection crises.

Anti-lymphocyte serum (ALS)

To damage lymphocytes by injecting an anti-lymphocyte serum was a nineteenth-century idea. Metchnikoff produced such a serum in 1899 and sixty years later Sir Michael Woodruff utilized this principle to produce immunosuppression. There is now extensive literature on the subject since ALS is an exceedingly powerful immunosuppressant in rodents. If mouse lymphocytes are injected repeatedly into rabbits, the rabbits become immunized. Blood from these animals is allowed to clot and the fluid remaining after the clot has been removed is called serum. This serum contains antibodies which will kill mouse lymphocytes. If this ALS is injected into mice they will often accept allografts indefinitely, sometimes they will also accept grafts from another species. Effective ALS has been produced between a variety of species, but with higher mammals and particularly primates it has proved to be more difficult to obtain powerful immunosuppressive sera without toxicity. If anti-dog ALS is prepared in the horse or rabbit, the sera contain powerful antibodies against red blood cells as well as lymphocytes and if injected into dogs, severe anaemia and dangerous allergic reactions may result. To prevent these complications the red cell antibodies must be absorbed before use by contact of the serum with dog red blood cells *in vitro*. Effective sera will then prolong the survival of allografts in dogs, but the resulting immunosuppression falls far short of that found with ALS in rodents.

Attempts have been made to remove ineffective and potentially dangerous protein from ALS. Analysis of the proteins has shown

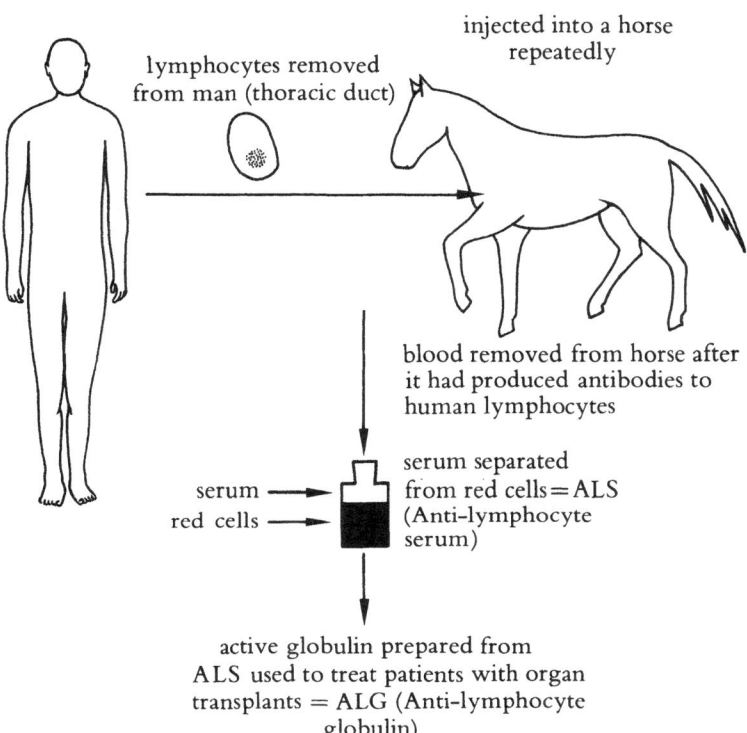

lymphocytes removed from man (thoracic duct)

injected into a horse repeatedly

blood removed from horse after it had produced antibodies to human lymphocytes

serum →
red cells →

serum separated from red cells = ALS (Anti-lymphocyte serum)

active globulin prepared from ALS used to treat patients with organ transplants = ALG (Anti-lymphocyte globulin)

FIG. 24. Diagram of the methods used to produce anti-lymphocyte serum (ALS) and anti-lymphocyte globulin (ALG). Human lymphocytes are injected into a horse which becomes immune to the human lymphocytes by producing antibodies in the serum. This serum is called anti-lymphocyte serum and is used as an immunosuppressive agent, being injected into patients with organ grafts. The anti-lymphocyte serum interferes with the immune response by damaging lymphocytes. Most of the activity of anti-lymphocyte serum is to be found in the purer and less toxic protein component called anti-lymphocyte globulin.

that most of the activity resides in the gamma globulins, which are the main antibody proteins. Anti-lymphocyte globulin (ALG) is therefore prepared for use in man. Fig. 24 shows the principle of ALG production for use in man. There is no doubt that ALG can be valuable in human organ transplantation. One of its most attractive properties is that it can be added to the standard Imuran and steroid regimen, thus increasing the immunosuppression without adding to the recognized toxic effects of these agents. ALG, however, has its own drawbacks. If injected under the skin or into muscle it can cause very severe local pain. If it is injected directly into the circulation it can cause allergic reactions with fever and *rigors*. There is also the possibility that the foreign protein may form complex aggregates which can damage the kidneys. ALS and ALG certainly destroy lymphocytes, but they may have other immunosuppressive actions. Routine clinical use has been delayed due to difficulties in obtaining a consistently effective product of known capabilities. Unfortunately no laboratory *in-vitro* test has yet been devised that can predict the *in-vivo* immunosuppressive activity. It is not known which species will produce the best ALS for use in man, although the horse has been favoured. Using the same lymphocyte injection schedules horses vary in their ability to produce ALS and an individual horse may provide ALS of varying and unpredictable properties at different times during the course of immunization. All sera require red blood cell absorption before use, but some also need to be absorbed with blood platelets to prevent a severe fall in the blood platelet count—thrombocytopaenia. To add to these difficulties, we do not yet know the optimal dose schedule for ALG treatment in man. Many of these problems will no doubt be solved and ALG may have an important part to play in clinical immunosuppression.

From the above consideration of immunosuppression it is obvious that our currently available agents are far from ideal. Toxic drugs and foreign protein injections are certainly not treatments of choice except as a last resort in an emergency situation. This unfortunately is the exact plight of a patient in need of a vital organ transplant, so until safer specific biological methods of immunosuppression become available, we must fall back on Imuran, steroids, and ALG.

CHAPTER FIVE

TISSUE MATCHING

In Chapter Three the inheritance of histocompatibility antigens that determine rejection was mentioned. Thus if a donor and recipient have exactly the same antigens, for example, identical twins or an inbred colony of mice, then grafts will not be rejected; in all other cases the presence of histocompatibility antigens in the donor, which are absent in the recipient, results in an immune rejection reaction after grafting. The aggressiveness of the reaction depends on the number and strength of the relevant incompatible antigens and also on the immune capabilities of the recipient. If the immune defences are weakened by the methods discussed in Chapter Four, then the response to all foreign antigens will be diminished; but for a given state of immune potential, the chances of a successful life-sustaining organ graft are inversely related to the number and strength of incompatible antigens. Thus when there is reasonably good compatibility, non-toxic doses of immuno-suppressive drugs will prevent rejection. Prior assessment of the incompatibility between donor and recipient is therefore desirable. Such an assessment is called tissue matching. A variety of techniques have been described, but only two have clinical relevance—namely serological tissue typing and *in-vitro* lymphocyte culture reactions.

SEROLOGICAL TISSUE TYPING

Histocompatibility antigens are present on all the cells of the body except red blood cells. The most convenient cells to use for typing are lymphocytes removed from a blood specimen. Red blood cell antigens are present in many other tissues besides red cells, and can therefore cause dangerous immune reactions. It is therefore important that these antigens are also determined. Red blood cell groups have been determined routinely for many years as an essential prerequisite to blood transfusion. The successful application of blood transfusion to medicine and surgery has saved countless lives, which are ample testimony to the importance of blood grouping. If a mistake is made and incompatible blood is transfused, dangerous reactions and even death may result due to destruction of the transfused red cells in the circulation. 'Typing' sera containing antibodies to the main A and B blood groups are readily available. Red blood cells from the individual whose blood is being grouped are mixed separately with anti-A and anti-B sera. If the relevant antigen is present in the red cells, they become clumped together. This agglutination therefore demonstrates incompatibility and also defines the red blood cell group as follows:

1. Red cells + anti-A serum ⟶ agglutination, therefore the patient's red cells contain A antigen.

2. Red cells + anti-B serum ⟶ agglutination, therefore the patient's red cells contain B antigen.

If an individual's red cells are agglutinated by anti-A serum, but not by anti-B, then that patient is group A. Conversely if the red cells are agglutinated by anti-B serum, but not by anti-A, the patient is group B. If the red cells are agglutinated by both anti-A and anti-B sera then the patient is group AB. If, however, the red cells are agglutinated by neither anti-A nor anti-B sera, then the patient is group O. It follows that red blood cells can be transfused from a group O donor to a recipient who is group O, A, B, or AB, since neither anti-A nor anti-B sera can agglutinate the group O red cells. Group O is, therefore, the universal blood donor group.

AB red blood cells will, however, be agglutinated by the sera of patients who are group O, A, or B since the serum of a group O patient has natural anti-A and anti-B antibodies, whilst the serum of a group A patient has anti-B antibodies and that of a group B patient has anti-A antibodies. AB red cells can therefore only be transfused to an AB recipient. From similar deductions it is clear that A red blood cells can be transfused into group A or AB recipients, but not into recipients of groups O or B, whilst B red cells can be transfused into group B or AB recipients, but not into recipients of groups A or O. It is apparent that AB recipients can safely receive red blood cells of any group. AB is, therefore, called the universal recipient group (Table I).

TABLE I

Red blood cells typing and transfusion

Donor blood group	Donor red cell antigen	Recipient blood group	Recipient serum antibody	Result of transfusion
A	A	A	anti-B	Satisfactory
	A	AB	nil	Satisfactory
	A	B	anti-A	Incompatible
	A	O	anti-A +anti-B	Incompatible
B	B	B	anti-A	Satisfactory
	B	AB	nil	Satisfactory
	B	A	anti-B	Incompatible
	B	O	anti-A +anti-B	Incompatible
O	O	AB	nil	Satisfactory
	O	A	anti-B	Satisfactory
	O	B	anti-A	Satisfactory
	O	O	anti-A +anti-B	Satisfactory
AB	AB	AB	nil	Satisfactory
	AB	A	anti-B	Incompatible
	AB	B	anti-A	Incompatible
	AB	O	anti-A +anti-B	Incompatible

The A and B antigen system is one of a complicated series of red blood cell groups. In the context of organ transplantation, however, A and B antigens are the only red cell antigens on organ grafts of sufficient strength to be important. Histocompatibility antigens as distinct from red cell antigens are numerous, complicated, and, at present, only partially understood. The principles of typing are, however, the same as for red cells. The test of incompatibility may be read as agglutination of blood lymphocytes or alternatively death of the lymphocytes—cytotoxicity. The techniques vary in detail but not in concept. Typing sera for histocompatibility antigens are not yet as clearly defined as are those for typing red cells. Histocompatibility antibodies develop in the sera of patients who have rejected tissue grafts, of patients who have had multiple blood transfusions, and of women who have had multiple pregnancies and have been immunized by their offspring. These sera are used to type lymphocytes of potential organ graft donors and recipients. If the lymphocytes of both donor and recipient are agglutinated or killed by a given typing serum, then as far as that serum is concerned the lymphocytes of both individuals have antigens in common. If they are not affected, then they lack antigens in common. If only the donor lymphocytes are affected, then the donor possesses an antigen that is absent in the recipient and vice versa. Careful analysis of the effects of numerous typing sera on the lymphocytes of related and unrelated individuals and correlation of these results with the subsequent behaviour of skin grafts has begun to clarify the nature of histocompatibility antigen inheritance and the relative strengths of different antigens. Most typing sera initially have antibodies against a number of antigens. Such multivalent sera are difficult and confusing to use. Removal of all but one of the antibodies, however, by selective absorption can provide monovalent sera which can detect and react with only one antigen. Specimens of a selection of different monovalent sera can then be distributed to tissue typing laboratories where the results of tissue typing will be comparable. This is of the utmost value in the practical utilization of tissue typing. Unfortunately, far more refined techniques will be required before serological typing can give an accurate prediction of the outcome of a graft in an individual case. Even with the present limitation, however, there is a definite statistical correlation of the number of mismatches between donor and recipient and the severity of rejection; but anomalies of severe rejection with a good match and vice versa are relatively frequent. Undoubtedly some of these cases are due to inadequate serological techniques, but another possibility is that serological typing gives no information on the immune potential of the recipient, which can be an important variable. Lymphocyte culture techniques may help in this assessment and they will now be discussed.

LYMPHOCYTE CULTURE REACTIONS

If blood lymphocytes from two individuals are cultured together in a nourishing medium they grow and divide. The proliferative activity can be assessed by measuring the incorporation of radio-active labelled materials by the cultured cells. This appears to be related to the degree of histo-incompatibility between the individuals. Thus lymphocyte proliferation can be regarded as an immune rejection reaction *in vitro*, and the intensity of this proliferation depends on the degree of mismatch between the lymphocytes. If the lymphocytes of the potential organ graft donor are prevented from reacting by treatment with X-rays, then the test becomes more useful as a laboratory model of the organ transplantation, since the recipient lymphocytes can mount an attack on defenceless donor cells (Fig. 25). The main disadvantage of this test is that it takes three to five days for the reaction to occur and therefore it can usually only be used with living kidney donors.

The practical application of tissue matching requires a twenty-four-hour service providing the specialized techniques. Potential

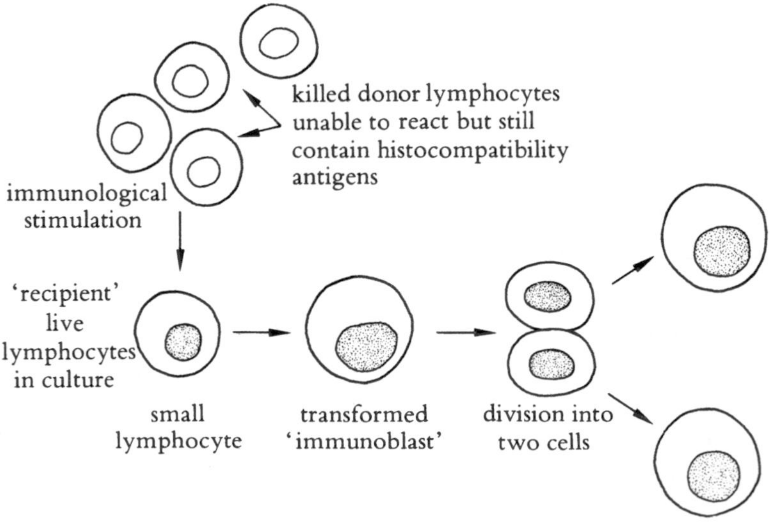

FIG. 25. Diagram of mixed lymphocyte culture reaction. This can be regarded as a laboratory model of an organ graft. The donor lymphocytes are killed to prevent them reacting by irradiation. However, their histocompatibility antigens are not damaged by this process. They are mixed in a nourishing culture fluid with normal non-irradiated recipient lymphocytes. Histocompatibility antigens present in the donor lymphocytes and absent in the recipient are recognized by the recipient lymphocytes which respond by enlarging and dividing. The degree of response is measured and gives an indication of the compatibility between donor and recipient. Thus, for example, if the lymphocytes came from identical twins there would be no reaction, whilst if donor and recipient are unrelated the chances are that a proliferating reaction would be observed, the severity of which will correlate with the fate of an organ transplanted from the same donor to the same recipient.

recipients of organ grafts are red cell grouped and tissue typed serologically as soon as they have been accepted into the transplantation programme. If kidney transplantation from a living donor is under consideration then the potential donor is similarly investigated and a mixed lymphocyte culture is set up as described above. There will be identity of tissue types and no mixed lymphocyte reaction between identical twins and occasionally between other closely related people. In random unrelated individuals, however, to find an identity of the known tissue groups is most unlikely and a mixed lymphocyte response of some degree is to be expected. The criteria of a relatively acceptable match are arbitrary and many factors require consideration. Important amongst these are the severity of the recipient's disease, the chances of keeping him alive to await an organ of a better match, the general availability of suitable organs, and the pressure on limited resources of other cases requiring treatment. These points will be considered later, but the objective, of course, will be to select the best possible match. With cadaver donors three to five days prior warning is unlikely, but serological typing can be accomplished in about three hours. It is, therefore, usually possible for this to be done before the death of the donor if there is sufficient warning, or immediately after the donor's death if the organ can be preserved for three hours. An important added precaution is to test the recipient's serum directly with donor lymphocytes. This 'cross match test' will detect preformed recipient antibodies that might otherwise have been missed. They may be the result of previous pregnancies, blood transfusions, or graft rejection, so it is particularly important to test for such antibodies in patients with a history of these conditions. To transplant a graft in the presence of antibodies that kill donor lymphocytes can result in immediate and disastrous hyperacute rejection of the transplant.

CHAPTER SIX

ORGAN PRESERVATION

The rapid deterioration of an organ deprived of its blood supply was referred to in Chapter Two. Individual organs differ in their susceptibility to ischaemic damage. Thus at normal body temperature the critical periods before irreversible destruction occurs are 3–5 minutes for the brain, 15–20 minutes for the liver, 30–40 minutes for the heart and lung, 50–100 minutes for the kidney, and up to 6 hours for skin and cornea. It is obviously desirable for the time lag between the onset of ischaemia and restoration of nourishment to the graft to be as short as possible, but excessive haste is unnecessary in removing the cornea for grafting, whilst every minute is of critical importance for a liver transplant. With a living kidney donor, elaborate preservation techniques are not used; instead, the operations on donor and recipient are synchronized so that the recipient is ready to receive the graft before the transplant is removed from the donor. Since restoration of a blood supply to the graft only takes 15–30 minutes, the kidney can be transplanted without cooling, but it is usually preferable to chill the organ. This can be done by immersing it in cold saline and/or infusing a cold physiological solution into the renal artery by gravity drainage from a blood transfusion drip-stand (Fig. 26). With cadaver donors, the kidneys are removed as soon as possible after death, preferably within one hour. The kidneys are then infused with cool solutions and kept cold at 4 °C in a refrigerator or surrounded by ice in a thermos flask. Meanwhile the recipient can

FIG. 26. Diagram showing simple cooling of a kidney which is placed in a dish surrounded by cold salt solution which cools its surface. Further cooling is provided by cold physiological fluid (1) run through a blood transfusion set into the renal artery (2). Once cold, the kidney is put into a sterile container which is surrounded by ice. It can then be transported cold in a thermos flask.

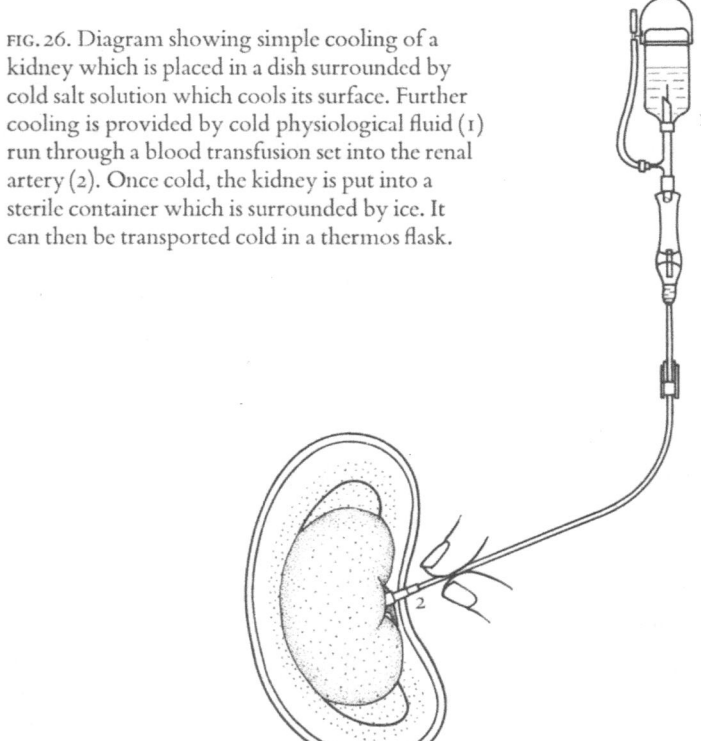

be prepared for operation and tissue typing of the donor can be performed, if this has not already been done. Kidneys prepared in this manner can be kept for 8–12 hours with little deterioration and they can be moved long distances during this period in a simple thermos flask. To keep a kidney for 12–72 hours a continuous perfusion apparatus is required. The principle here is to provide the organ with an artificial circulation, of cool oxygenated physiological solutions (Fig. 27). This type of organ preservation contains complicated bulky machinery with the disadvantages that there are risks of electrical or mechanical faults developing. There is also a serious hazard that infective bacteria may gain access to the

ORGAN PRESERVATION

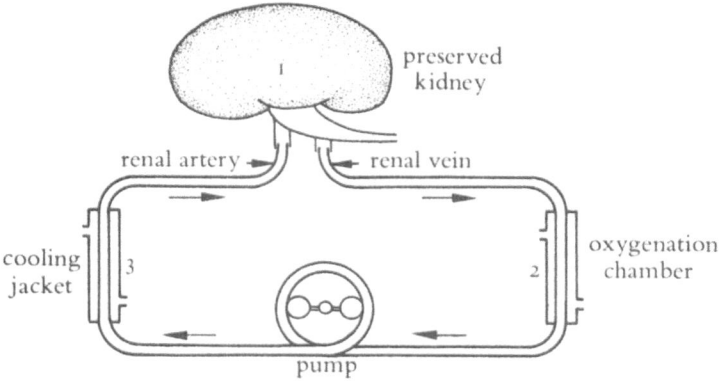

FIG. 27. Diagram of organ preservation by continuous cold perfusion. The organ being preserved, a kidney (1) is protected within a sterile container. Physiological fluid is oxygenated (2), cooled (3), and pumped into the renal artery. The effluent from the renal vein completing the circuit.

perfusion circulation and then be transferred with the graft to the recipient. There is slow deterioration of organs undergoing continuous mechanical perfusion that does not occur *in vivo* and attempts to keep organs in a well-preserved state for much longer than 72 hours have failed. Although blood cells, spermatozoa, and certain other dissociated cells can be kept alive indefinitely at subzero temperatures, the preserving fluids, that prevent cell destruction by ice crystals, have toxic effects if introduced into whole organs like the kidney. There are no signs of an imminent solution to long-term organ storage.

The time limits of preservation by cooling alone and cooling with continuous perfusion have not been as extensively studied for the heart, lung, and liver as for the kidney. The principles are the same but these organs are less tolerant of ischaemic damage. A very important practical difference between the kidney and other vital organs is that reversible ischaemic damage, which temporarily interferes with function, is not a disaster following kidney transplantation, since the patient can be maintained by dialysis. There is no equivalent safety feature to tide patients over with grafts of heart, lung, and liver. These organs must function well immediately after operation otherwise the patient will die. It is possible to remove the heart or lung immediately after death and transplant them successfully without cooling, but the increased safety margin of simple chilling is preferred by most surgeons. Since the liver suffers irreversible damage without its blood supply after more than 15–20 minutes at 37 °C and removal and transplantation of the liver are complicated and time-consuming procedures, it is obligatory to cool the organ. Three techniques have been used:

1. Cooling and perfusing the whole corpse with a heart–lung machine. Blood is drained from the femoral vein in the groin, it is cooled and oxygenated by the machine, and then pumped into the femoral artery, whence it passes to all organs of the body and cools them. This procedure requires complicated machinery which must be readily available, and even with skilled surgery there will be 5–10 minutes delay whilst the femoral vessels are cannulated before the perfusion can be started.

2. Infusion of cold physiological fluid into the portal vein to cool the liver before it is removed. This can be started within 5 minutes of death and is simple (Fig. 28). The cold infusion is continued until the liver is removed. The organ is then placed in a sterile plastic bag which is surrounded by an ice and water mixture. This will maintain the liver in a healthy state for about 4 hours, during which time the transplant operation must be completed.

3. To keep a liver more than 4 hours it is necessary to provide it with an artificial circulation by continuous perfusion. The most successful apparatus, so far designed, pumps diluted cold blood through the liver. The perfusate is oxygenated under high pressure. The disadvantages of this type of apparatus have been mentioned, but it can allow 4 hours additional preservation time compared with simple cooling.

ORGAN PRESERVATION

Current methods of preserving organs fall far short of the ideal of an 'organ bank'. Many difficulties must be overcome before we can keep organs in the same way that blood is banked.

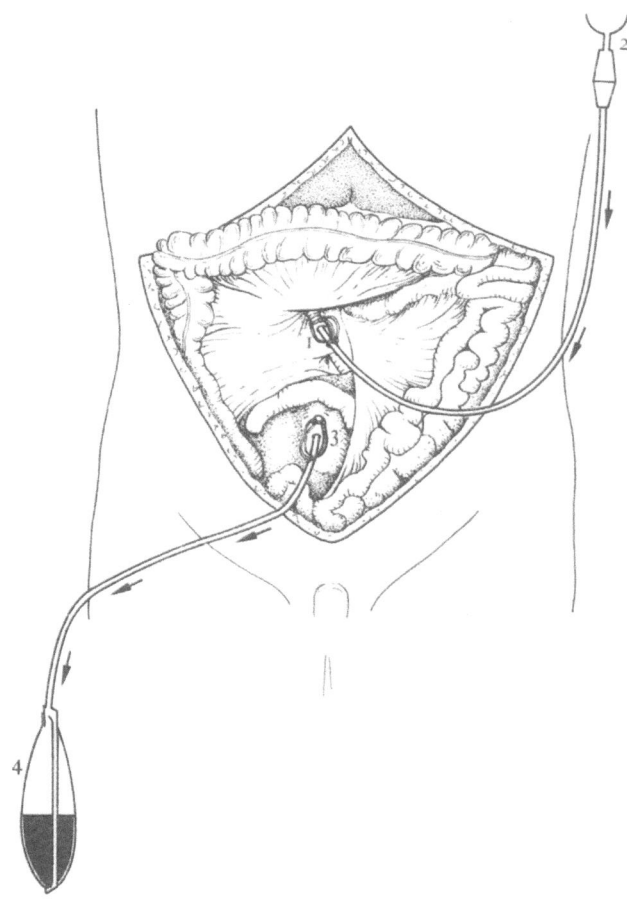

FIG. 28. Diagram of a simple method used to cool the liver immediately after death. A physiological solution is run into the portal vein (1) through a blood transfusion drip set (2). At the same time the inferior vena cava (3) is decompressed with a cannula draining into a plastic bag (4). This prevents congestion of the liver. This cooling continues whilst the liver is being removed. (By courtesy of the *British Journal of Surgery*)

CHAPTER SEVEN

SUITABLE DONORS

Tissue matching was discussed in Chapter Five and ethical factors will be considered in Chapter Nine. In this chapter I will describe the suitability of donors from the point of view of biological function unrelated to the possibilities of rejection. A perfectly functioning kidney graft should result if the donor is healthy and alive when the kidney is removed. Opinions differ on the criteria that should be established in selection of living donors. If the potential donor is over 21, a blood relation of the recipient of a compatible red blood cell group, and a good tissue match, then I feel serious consideration should be given to his declared wish to donate a kidney. Removal of one kidney from a healthy person is a painful major operation with a small but definite risk to life. Although survival into old age is possible with one kidney, injury to or disease of the one remaining kidney will obviously constitute a threat to life that would not exist if there were two kidneys. It is first necessary to confirm that the volunteer kidney donor is healthy. In particular he must not be suffering from any infectious or malignant condition and his blood pressure should be normal. His urine is then examined for any abnormal constituents and his kidneys and urinary drainage tract are X-rayed after injection into a vein of radio-opaque material which is excreted by the kidneys. This intravenous pyelogram gives information on kidney function and, most important, shows that two normal kidneys are present. The arteries of the kidneys are also X-rayed by injecting into them radio-opaque solution using a flexible catheter inserted via the femoral artery in the groin. Multiple renal arteries are common and can prejudice the surgical success of a transplant operation. If this rather rigorous assessment is satisfactory and careful explanation of all the hazards, the pain and discomfort of having a kidney removed have not deterred the donor from his wish, then I feel it the duty of transplantation surgeons is to proceed. Of course, there are many features that may be important in an individual decision, and transplantation surgeons vary in their rules of selection. I think it is most important to try to exclude any possibility that pressure is being exerted on the 'donor' by other members of his family, or that he is motivated merely by a sense of duty or guilt if he refuses. There should be an obvious and genuine wish to donate his kidney, in fact a feeling that he will have been deprived if his request is refused.

What should be the policy for those under 21 years and volunteer donors who are not blood relations? I would be most reluctant to take a kidney for transplantation from a child, but exactly at what age to draw the line would depend on the degree of understanding of the individual. For example, a normal 18-year-old identical twin could be an acceptable donor since the emotional ties of identical twins are so close and the anticipated result of the transplant is excellent. On the other hand, I would not consider a child donor of 10 years as suitable even if the potential recipient was his mother or a brother or sister, since full comprehension of the situation is not possible at 10 years. I am not prepared to transplant from live donors who are not blood relations, even if the would-be donor is a spouse, since the anticipated results are no better than those of cadaver donors. In any individual case the decision may be difficult and involve numerous discussions with many people. Suitable live donors are rather unusual since so many criteria, both medical and social, must be satisfied. In a consecutive series of 100 kidney transplants performed in Cambridge, only 4 were from living donors.

The most suitable cadaver donor for any organ transplant should have been previously healthy before the terminal illness. The cause of death should not have been associated with infection, malignancy, or prolonged low blood pressure. Infection or malignancy may be spread to the recipient by the graft. Prolonged low blood pressure interferes with the circulation and, therefore, the nourishment of vital organs. These stipulations include most patients dying in hospital from being organ donors. Suitable donors will have died from accidents, particularly head injuries, primary brain tumours, which do not spread outside the skull, sudden brain haemorrhages or thrombosis, and coronary thrombosis—this last disease, of course, precludes use of the heart for transplantation. In fact, if a suitable donor heart was available some cases of coronary thrombosis might benefit from receiving a heart graft. This unsavoury suggestion of priorities would not exist in practice, since if there was any chance of saving the life of a patient dying of coronary thrombosis this chance would be taken, even if this meant cardiac transplantation. The possibility of the patient being an organ donor would only arise after irreversible brain damage had occurred, despite every effort having been made to provide the best treatment.

The age of a donor does not seem to be of great importance except with regard to the size of the organ to be transplanted. Thus organs from children or the elderly can be used if the circumstances of death were as specified. Gross size discrepancy may, however, preclude successful surgery, for example, an adult's liver cannot be grafted into a child, but the reverse is possible and children's livers have been successfully transplanted into adults. A small child's heart would not be able to maintain the circulation in an adult even if the surgery could be accomplished. Organs from the very old may have suffered from degenerative changes and, therefore, be unsuitable as grafts. Infants shortly after birth have a low blood pressure and even if their organs could be transplanted with potential function they might suffer irreversible damage from sudden exposure to an unaccustomed higher blood pressure.

Although many deaths exclude the possibility of organ donation, there are more than enough satisfactory donors to graft all patients requiring kidney and liver transplantation, if only use could be made of all suitable cases. The indications for heart and lung transplantation are not yet fully defined, so it is not possible to determine whether there would be sufficient donor organs. Some published predictions of the numbers of transplants that might be performed if rejection could be controlled seem to me to be excessive. The use of gross statistics of deaths from heart and lung disease do not give sufficient information on other relevant factors, such as the time available to prepare for the operation and perform the transplantation before the patient would die. In patients with heart and lung illness there may also be serious disease in other organs which would preclude transplantation.

CHAPTER EIGHT

TRANSPLANTATION OF INDIVIDUAL ORGANS

In this chapter I will briefly summarize certain features of grafts of the kidney, liver, heart, and lung that have not yet been considered.

THE KIDNEY

This was the first organ to be successfully transplanted in man. The surgery is straightforward. Dialysis allows the patient to be reasonably fit whilst awaiting operation and can keep him in health if the organ is slow to function. Experience of kidney transplantation in man is now considerable, but since effective immunosuppression has only been available for nine years it is too early to predict how long a kidney transplant might function. Fatal kidney disease is quite common and young adults are particularly liable to be affected. Out of a population of some 50 million in England and Wales, there are 2,000–3,000 deaths from kidney disease each year in patients between 5 and 55 years of age. The three diseases responsible for most of these deaths affect both kidneys equally and progressively. They are glomerulonephritis or Bright's disease, pyelonephritis due to chronic kidney infection and, less common, polycystic disease, an inherited abnormality of the kidneys in which slow deterioration of function of the kidneys usually results in death in the fourth or fifth decade.

When all available conventional treatment has been given, yet deterioration of renal function continues, the patient eventually becomes anaemic and weak. He may be unable to excrete water and as a result extra fluid collecting in the tissues produces dropsy or oedema. Fluid accumulation in the lungs may cause difficulty in breathing and put an excessive strain on the heart, which is liable to be under strain already from high blood pressure, a common accompaniment of kidney failure. The retained waste products build up in the body and can cause inflammation of the external lining of the heart and the inner lining of the colon and stomach. Pericarditis may cause chest pain, colitis, diarrhoea, and gastritis, one of the most distressing features of renal failure—persistent vomiting. The limb nerves may cease to function—this peripheral neuritis can paralyse the muscles and prevent the patient from moving. This tragic picture of renal failure or uraemia is exceedingly unpleasant for the patient and distressing to his relatives. For the doctor and nurses caring for a patient dying from uraemia, the sadness and frustration are particularly poignant, since they are well aware of the fact that combined treatment of dialysis and kidney grafting could cure all the symptoms, and there would be a good chance of restoring the patient to a normal or nearly normal existence. Yet only a minority, less than 10 per cent of uraemic patients, will receive adequate treatment. This is due mainly to a shortage of donor kidneys that could easily be available if there was more understanding and co-operation in the community and within the medical profession.

There is no satisfactory method of selecting who should be treated. In fact it is an indictment of our community to raise the question, since a National Health Service should provide the best treatment available to all, irrespective of any personal considerations. Arguments that the financial burden would be overwhelming are entirely spurious. The folly and extent of wastage of treasury funds is not germane to my theme and, in any case, the target is too large to be worth shooting at. Specifically in relation to the treatment of renal disease, however, it is not difficult to construct a sound financial argument. To treat a uraemic patient in hospital until he dies costs approximately £50 per week, and the stay in hospital may last three months or more, which is a period of suffering for the patient, with death at the end and personal tragedy for the family. To restore a patient to health and a job is an economic asset to the State and the hospital costs involved in this treatment are unlikely to be greatly in excess of the negative alternative. The Department of Health in the United Kingdom has recognized the need to treat uraemic patients and has invested considerable sums in establishing regional dialysis and transplantation units, but these units cannot operate if shortage of donor kidneys prevent progress of patients through the units, since the beds will become blocked. Until the situation improves the only tolerable way of accepting patients is on a strict waiting-list basis, in the bitter knowledge that most patients will die before they can be admitted, due to lack of available beds in the dialysis and transplantation units.

Once admitted, the patient is blood grouped, tissue typed, screened for cytotoxic antibodies, and a plastic Scribner shunt is inserted or an arterio-venous Brescia–Cimino fistula is constructed so that haemodialysis can be started (Figs. 29 and 30). The Scribner shunt is convenient to use, but has the disadvantage that clotting or infection may occur where the plastic joins the blood vessels. The U-tube is opened and the two cannulas joined to the kidney machine when the patient is dialysed (Fig. 31). After dialysis the tube is reconnected and the fast flow of blood directly from artery to vein tends to prevent the shunt from clotting. When clots do occur they can sometimes be removed from the shunt, but even with great care it is unusual for a shunt to last more than one year. Every time a new shunt is inserted the limited number of available arteries and veins in the arms and legs become reduced and eventually all the shunt sites may be used up. The Brescia–Cimino

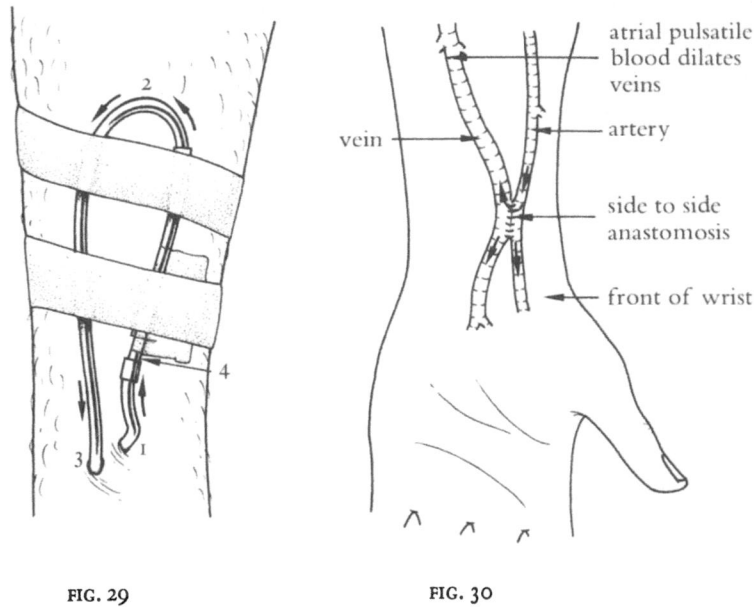

atrial pulsatile
blood dilates
veins

vein

artery

side to side
anastomosis

front of wrist

FIG. 29   FIG. 30

FIG. 29. Diagram of a 'Scribner shunt' used for repeated haemodialysis. A plastic cannula (1) is inserted into an artery joined by a U-tube (2) to another plastic cannula (3), which is inserted into a vein. As shown in the diagram, blood passes from the artery around the U-tube into the vein. When the patient is treated by the artificial kidney the tube is disconnected at the point marked (4) on the diagram, and the two lines are joined to the artificial kidney so that blood goes from the artery into the artificial kidney and back into the vein. At the end of the treatment the U-tube is reconnected.

FIG. 30. Diagram of Brescia–Cimino fistula used for repeated haemodialysis. A surgical anastomosis is performed between an artery and vein in the arm. As a result blood under high pressure in the artery passes into the vein and dilates all the veins of the arm, which stand up prominently under the skin. When the patient is to receive artificial kidney treatment a needle is passed into one of these veins, blood is sucked off and pumped into the artificial kidney machine and back via another needle, which is inserted into a different vein.

consol containing concentrate of chemicals
which is mixed with water to make a
physiological solution at body temperature

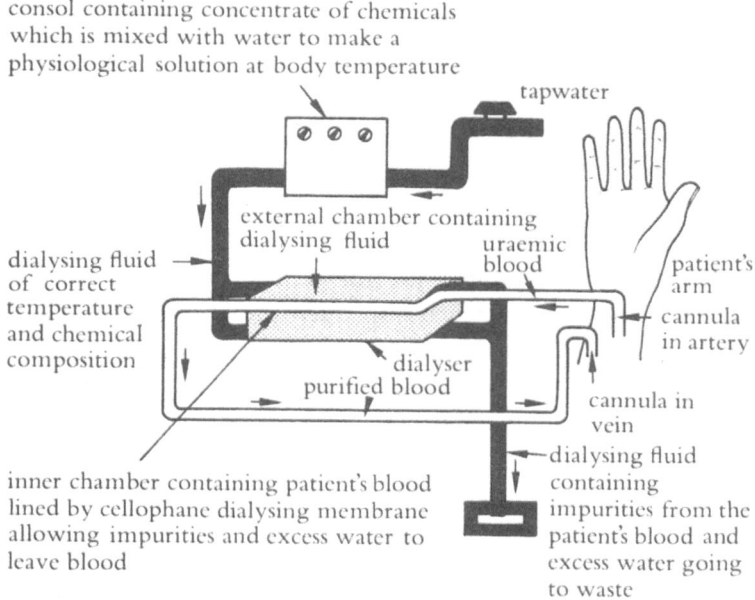

tapwater

external chamber containing
dialysing fluid

uraemic
blood

dialysing fluid
of correct
temperature
and chemical
composition

patient's
arm

cannula
in artery

dialyser
purified blood

cannula in
vein

inner chamber containing patient's blood
lined by cellophane dialysing membrane
allowing impurities and excess water to
leave blood

dialysing fluid
containing
impurities from the
patient's blood and
excess water going
to waste

FIG. 31. Diagram of haemodialysis. Blood is taken from a Scribner shunt or a
Brescia–Cimino fistula. It passes into the artificial kidney machine within the
dialysing membrane. On the other side of the membrane is physiological fluid.
Whilst in contact with the membrane impurities in the blood pass into the
dialysing fluid. Essential constituents lacking in the patient pass from the dialysing fluid into the blood and the purified blood then returns to the patient's vein.

fistula is a direct surgical anastomosis of a small artery to a vein.
After one to two weeks the rapid flow of blood at high pressure in
the vein causes all the veins of the limb to dilate. Every time the
patient is dialysed a large needle is inserted into a dilated pulsating
vein and blood pumped from the vessel through the needle into the
dialysis machine and returned via a needle in another vein. These
fistula seldom clot or become infected, but repeated needling can
cause discomfort and requires skill.

After a few weeks of dialysis for fourteen hours two to three
times a week, all features of uraemia diminish and the patient can

usually get out of bed and regain his strength. Full assessment can then be made of the best policy of management. There can be no doubt that a patient with a good transplant feels better and is far more independent than a patient whose life depends on dialysis two to three times a week. The best chance of a good transplant is early after the onset of uraemia, since repeated dialysis with the occasional need for blood transfusion can sensitize the patient and produce cytotoxic antibodies that may reject a transplant. In addition the sooner a patient is transplanted the quicker the dialysis space becomes vacant so that another patient may be treated. Provided the patient is considered to be medically suitable for a transplant, as soon as he is fit for operation, both his diseased kidneys are removed. There are three main reasons for removing both kidneys (bilateral nephretomy).

1. If the kidneys are infected then a dangerous bacterial focus is removed. Even if they are not infected beforehand, after successful transplantation they may become infected when the patient is treated with immunosuppressive drugs.

2. Diseased kidneys often cause dangerous high blood pressure by producing a hypertensive agent called renin. Removal of the kidneys usually helps control the blood pressure.

3. The removed kidneys can be examined and errors in the diagnosis of the kidney disease can be avoided. In particular, if the disease is a very active glomerulonephritis, direct study of the diseased kidney may show whether it is likely that the disease might affect a transplant, in which case kidney grafting would be contra-indicated.

If there are no complicating factors, as soon as the patient has recovered from the bilateral nephrectomy he will be ready for grafting either from a live donor or a cadaver. After the operation, if the kidney came from a cadaver, dialysis may be required for two to three weeks whilst reversible ischaemic damage is repaired. The patient is given Imuran and steroids. Anti-lymphocyte globulin is added if a good preparation is available. For the first ten days after the operation, before the wound is fully healed, the patient is nursed in a room in which efforts are made to exclude bacteria. The room is cleaned frequently and receives pressure ventilation with filtered air. Doctors, nurses, and close relatives, who visit the patient, wash carefully and wear masks and gowns. After ten days the patient is encouraged to be up and about as much as possible. During the first four months after surgery most complications occur, the commonest being rejection of the graft and infection. Surveillance of the patient during this time must be particularly careful. The patient is discharged from hospital as soon as possible after operation, sometimes this may be as early as three weeks, but more often it is about six weeks. Frequent monitoring of kidney function and the bone marrow is necessary, so that the correct dosage of immunosuppressive agents can be given to each individual. According to changes in the observations so treatment may need adjusting. If the graft is functioning well with a stable dose of immunosuppression, the patient is encouraged to return to work. The quality of life can be almost normal, the only restrictions being the necessity to take tablets daily and attend hospital at regular intervals for medical assessment. In fact the restrictions are less severe than those imposed on most patients with diabetes, since diabetics need a special diet and insulin has to be injected. Both Imuran and steroids are taken by mouth and ALG is not normally continued after discharge from hospital. Patients with kidney grafts can do a full day's work; one of our patients has been a bulldozer driver after receiving his graft. Men can become fathers and women can bear normal children. If the transplant is rejected, or fails for some other reason, such as infection, immunosuppressive drugs are stopped, the graft is removed and the patient returned to maintenance dialysis. There are now three alternative possibilities:

1. Regular dialysis may be continued indefinitely in hospital or on an out-patient basis. This should be avoided if possible, since a dialysis space is blocked permanently. 2. It is far preferable to transplant a second kidney or 3, teach the patient to dialyse himself at home. If there are no cytotoxic antibodies, most patients after recovering from the previous operation would prefer a second graft in which the chances of success are unlikely to be severely prejudiced by the first transplant (Fig. 32). If, however, cytotoxic antibodies are present in the serum, it may take a long time to find a suitable donor, in which the direct 'cross-match' test is negative

FIG. 32. Mr. K. J. two years after receiving a second transplant from a dead donor, the first one having failed after eleven days. The patient is in good health and is able to work normally as a mechanic.

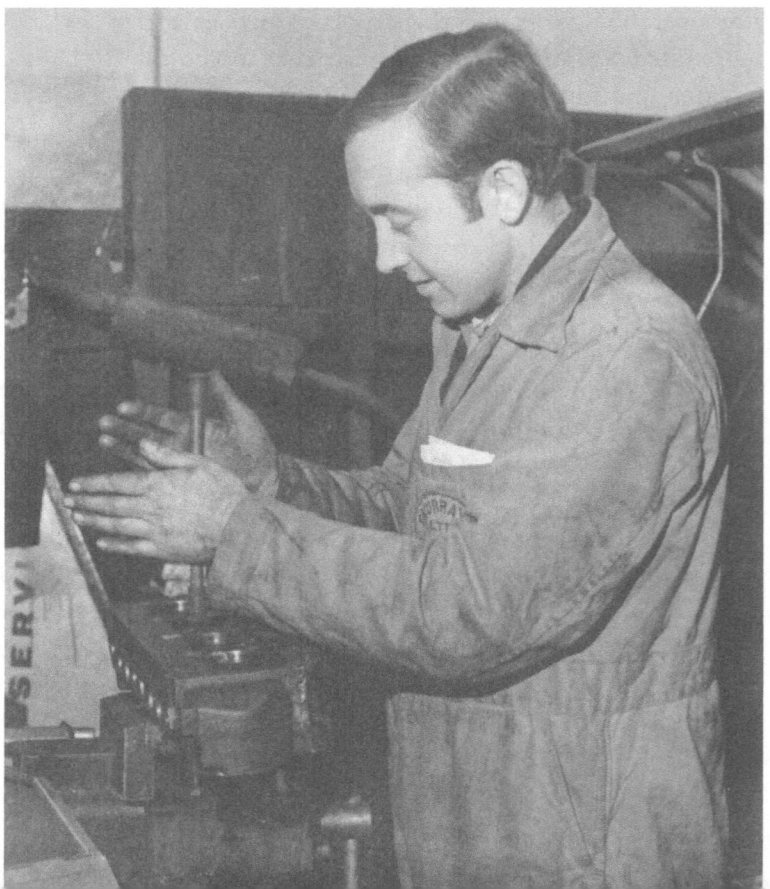

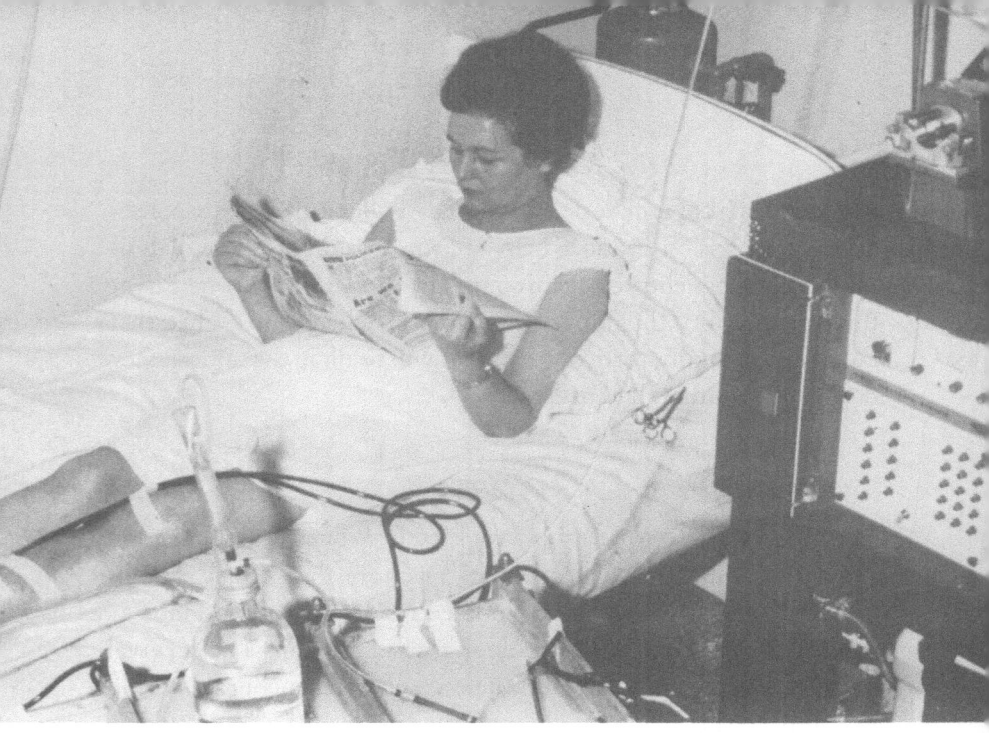

FIG. 33. Patient on dialysis in her own home. She started treatment in April 1965 and is in good health. All the equipment fits into quite a small area in her house. (By courtesy of Dr. Stanley Shaldon)

and dialysis at home may be preferable at least for a time. After adequate instruction, home dialysis is well within the technical capabilities of most people of normal intelligence (Fig. 33). Some patients, however, are not able to cope because of psychological difficulties. Prolonged dependence on the hospital and the disappointment of a failed operation may understandably make home dialysis a frightening prospect. Transplantation and dialysis units will, as time goes on, accumulate more and more patients who are untransplantable yet unwilling to dialyse themselves. This may prove to be a very serious problem that could undermine the whole scheme of treatment for irreversible kidney disease. If one out of twenty patients originally admitted became wedded to continued hospital dialysis, it would only be a few years before all hospital dialysis space was occupied. It is necessary for more attention to be

paid to this problem, otherwise there will be disastrous conse-
quences. Provision of more help and supervision of home dialysis
might allow patients to regain confidence and eventually take over
the responsibility themselves, particularly when they realize that
failure to accept this form of treatment will result in the unnecessary
deaths of the other patients.

RESULTS

Dr. Murray in Boston set up a registry of kidney transplantation
operations which has collected data on more than 2,000 patients
from all over the world. These pooled results give a good indication of the present status of kidney transplantation. The survival
data are shown in Table II. These results are encouraging and
certainly compare favourably with the results of the best available
treatment for many forms of cancer. The short period during

TABLE II

Results of 2,347 kidney transplants

Donor	Survival		Longest
	1 year	*2 years*	*surviving*
Identical twin 1%	91%	89%	12 years
Blood relatives 48%	87%	77%	10 years
Cadaver 51%	42%	40%	5 years

which kidney transplantation has been practised makes long-term
assessment impossible. We do not know if a transplant can give a
young patient a full life-span, nevertheless if anyone has any doubts
of the general value of this form of treatment for young adults, I
can assure them that these doubts are not shared by the patients
themselves. To be restored from a uraemic death to a normal life

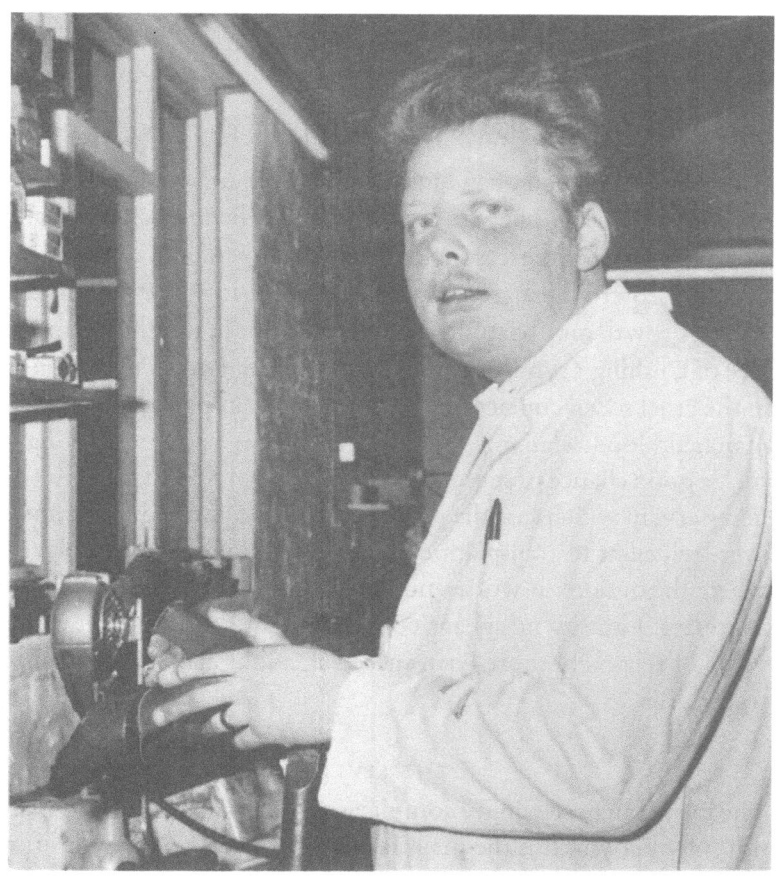

FIG. 34. **Mr. J. L.** at work more than four years after receiving a kidney transplant from a dead donor. When admitted to hospital this patient was paralysed, vomiting continuously, and in a moribund state.

with a functioning graft is considered to be well worth while by most patients, even if the benefit is as short-lived as six months—and more than a year of extra life, if this is full and enjoyable, entirely justifies the procedure (Fig. 34). The results now obtained make it possible to offer nearly an 80 per cent chance of two years' survival, with a well-matched graft from a blood relative and a 40 per cent chance of two-year survival with an unmatched cadaver transplant. Moreover, should the transplant fail it may be removed and the patient maintained by dialysis or re-transplanted.

ORGAN TRANSPLANTS

I am not so certain of the justification of kidney transplantation for young children. They are unable to comprehend the situation and cannot understand the reasons for dialysis, an operation, and repeated injections. Steroid drugs produce more side-effects in children than adults: growth may be stunted and the increase in weight and moon face of Cushing's syndrome may cause the child much unhappiness in the cruel social contacts of the young. A transplant from a well-matched blood relative, which usually means a parent, may have such a good chance of success that high doses of steroids may not be necessary, in which case the procedure may be justified. I am, however, reluctant to transplant children with kidneys from cadavers where the outlook is worse and the likelihood of high steroid dose is greater. I am by no means convinced that the argument of the value of relatively short-term success in adults can also be applied to children.

THE LIVER

The liver is an exceedingly complicated organ, whose functions are not fully known. It is the main factory of the body. It obtains raw materials in the form of amino acids, the building bricks of proteins and other metabolites, via its private blood supply, the portal vein. This carries absorbed nourishment from the intestines to the liver. The liver manufactures a whole variety of essential proteins which include the blood clotting factors and serum albumin. In addition it converts bile pigment from broken-down red cells into a chemical form that it can excrete. This, together with bile salts, which aid fat digestion, constitute bile which passes via the gall bladder and bile duct into the duodenum. The liver also plays an essential part in the regulation of sugar metabolism. If the liver fails, the blood sugar level can fall so low that coma results. The liver detoxifies potentially poisonous products of metabolism and intestinal absorption. If it fails to remove certain nitrogen-containing protein derivatives of digestion, these pass into the main systemic blood stream and cause derangement of the brain and coma (porto-systemic encephalopathy).

There are two categories of fatal liver disease which can be treated by liver transplantation, namely primary cancer of the liver cells or bile ducts and non-malignant diseases of the liver cells, for example, cirrhosis of the liver. In this disease the damaged liver is invaded with fibrous tissue which strangle its blood supply and leads to the death of liver cells and blockage of the portal vein. High pressure in the portal vein may produce varicose veins of the gullet which are liable to catastrophic and often lethal bleeding. In the United Kingdom the cause of most cases of cirrhosis is unknown, although the disease can follow severe infective hepatitis or alcoholism. Alcoholism is a common cause of cirrhosis on the continent of Europe and in North America. Cirrhosis can also follow obstruction of the flow of bile. Biliary cirrhosis in which jaundice is a marked feature can occur in adults, but is commoner and particularly tragic in infants, who are born without bile ducts. Children with this condition usually die in the first or second year of life and no treatment can help them. Another type of liver disease in children that might become a suitable indication for liver transplantation is congenital deficiency of certain vital liver enzymes, whose absence prevent the liver from functioning normally and early death results. Acute fatal liver damage from poisoning or virus infection might also be treated by liver transplantation. The number of young people dying from liver disease in Britain is probably about 10 per cent of the incidence of fatal kidney disease; that is, approximately 200–300 deaths a year. In some parts of the world, particularly the Far East, the incidence is much higher.

Dr. Moore and his colleagues in Boston and Dr. Starzl's group in Denver evolved satisfactory techniques of orthotopic liver transplantation in dogs. Laboratory studies led directly to clinical application in which the outstanding worker has been Dr. Starzl. It has proved to be very difficult to obtain good results for a variety of reasons which will now be considered.

1. The poor condition of the recipient

It is not justifiable to consider a new and dangerous form of therapy until all conventional treatments have been tried and have failed. When it is then clear that the patient is dying and is not well enough to lead an existence outside of hospital, then it is reasonable to offer a new and risky operation. Most patients are anxious for the chance, since the alternative is certain death. The doctors are not involved in callous experimentation but are genuinely concerned to find new ways of saving life and diminishing suffering. The new treatment is based on extensive investigation in animals, but it is well known that although the results of animal experimentation usually suggest a parallel response in man, there can be no guarantee that the findings in one species will apply to another. Eventually a cautious, carefully studied human trial must be undertaken of encouraging methods developed in the laboratory.

In the early stages of a new operation there is a tendency to operate on patients who are moribund and are unlikely to withstand the extensive surgery. If, however, there is even a minute chance of success and the patient and relatives wish the operation to be attempted then it is justifiable to proceed. Although there will be many failures, occasional success represents a valuable gain, since without operation the patient would be dead. This principle is not new in surgery. In fact it is daily surgical practice to try to save the seemingly hopeless case—for instance, massive bleeding from a ruptured aorta, severe haemorrhage from a peptic ulcer, and rupture of obstructed bowel. Many further examples could be stated.

I feel it is important to realize this surgical principle since it explains the disappointing results of early attempts at new operations, which eventually become standard practice. When the mortality becomes acceptably low it is justifiable for surgery to be undertaken at an early stage in the disease. This was the pattern of development of kidney transplantation; in fact, nine years ago the results of kidney transplantation were worse than those now obtained with liver and heart grafts. There is, however, one important difference to which reference has already been made, namely the remarkable benefits of dialysis for kidney failure for which there is no equivalent in other vital organ diseases. Acute liver failure has occasionally been successfully treated by temporary substitution of liver function over a critical period whilst the liver recovers. Three methods have been used:

1. Exchanging the patient's blood for fresh blood from donors with normal liver function. Vast quantities of blood may be required, far more than the maximum likely requirement in liver transplantation, yet results are poor, probably inferior to those of a liver graft.

2. Passage of the patient's blood through an animal's liver or human cadaver liver outside the body. Temporary improvement often follows such an *ex-vivo* liver perfusion, but the procedure cannot be repeated indefinitely and relapse speedily follows cessation of treatment.

3. Cross-circulation of the patient's blood with a human volunteer or an animal—for example, a baboon. This form of treatment can also be temporarily effective, but there is considerable risk to a human donor and animal antigens may cause dangerous reactions in the patient if the procedure is repeated.

None of these methods can restore a patient dying of liver disease to a satisfactory state of health to withstand a major operation. They are in no way comparable to dialysis for kidney failure.

2. *The paucity of suitable donors*

All the difficulties of obtaining donors that were mentioned in relation to the kidney apply to the liver, but with the liver the problems are greatly increased. It was explained that to be of value for transplantation the liver must be cooled within fifteen minutes of death, and then can be kept safely for only four hours in the cold or eight hours if subjected to complicated continuous perfusion. To proceed with liver transplantation it is necessary for the transplantation team to have prior warning of the likelihood of a suitable donor since the surgical preparations are complicated. The best results are obtained in cases in which resuscitation has been attempted but has failed and where, for reasons unconnected with transplantation, a decision has been made to abandon artificial support of breathing and the circulation. It is then possible to cool the liver within the critical time after death. Such cases are, however, unusual and many potential recipients die of their liver disease before a transplant can be found.

3. *Operative difficulties*

The rather complicated anatomy of the liver has already been mentioned. Both removal of the liver from a corpse and its grafting into the recipient are technically exacting, but the surgery is well-established and no surgeon would attempt this operation in man without first gaining an extensive experience in animals. In the human patient, however, there are additional problems not encountered in animals. The most important difference is in the removal of the diseased liver in the recipient. Excision of a huge diseased liver can be a formidable undertaking, particularly if the liver pathology has blocked the portal venous circulation and caused portal hypertension. The patient will usually have had previous abdominal surgery to establish a diagnosis or treat the liver condition. This previous surgery will have caused adhesions between the liver and its surroundings and the intestines. The adhesions are likely to be vascular and, if the portal blood pressure is high, there may be multiple abnormal thin-walled blood vessels which tend to bleed profusely. This bleeding tendency is aggravated by the lack of clotting factors resulting from poor liver function. Thus recipient hepatectomy can be troublesome and rapid blood loss needs to be speedily replaced to prevent the patient from becoming shocked, since grafting of a perfect liver to a shocked patient will be of no avail because the low blood pressure will be insufficient to perfuse and nourish the transplant, which will therefore not function. No new clotting factors will be produced and further bleeding will occur. A vicious circle is set up with increasing shock, liver failure, haemorrhage, and death. This same sequence of events follows grafting a poorly preserved liver that has suffered ischaemic damage, into a patient who is not shocked, since the failure of the damaged liver to produce clotting factors leads to uncontrollable haemorrhage and shock. On the other hand, grafting a well-preserved liver to a non-shocked patient has the immensely gratifying result of new clotting factor production and a rapid and dramatic cessation of operative bleeding and good liver function. This is the only satisfactory outcome of a liver transplant operation.

4. *Post-operative factors*

If the patient is to survive the operation, the liver must function immediately and continue with good function, for there is little supportive management possible and no leeway comparable to that provided by dialysis after kidney grafts. Otherwise management is similar, the same immunosuppressive agents are used, but Imuran is potentially toxic to the liver and the dose has to be monitored carefully and assessed in relation to liver function. Rejection leads to liver failure which may be acute or slow and insidious. Recurrence of the patient's original disease has only so far been observed when the liver pathology was cancer. The disease had not been eradicated at the time of surgery and must have spread outside the liver and grown in different parts of the body after the transplant operation, eventually spreading to the grafted liver itself. The incidence of this complication had not yet been established.

With this background it is perhaps not surprising that many liver transplantation operations have led to disappointment and failure, but the procedure is certainly possible and capable of providing valuable therapy in patients otherwise doomed. Dr. Starzl has had several patients survive more than one year and has even successfully transplanted a second liver after the first had failed. Two of our patients are at home and well eleven months and one year after orthotopic liver grafting (Figs. 35 and 36). Their livers functioned

FIG. 35. Mr. G. K. after removal of his own liver and transplantation of a liver from a dead donor. This patient was in coma prior to the operation, due to his liver disease. After the operation he recovered immediately from the coma and is now very well eleven months after receiving the liver graft. (By courtesy of the Editor of the *Daily Telegraph*)

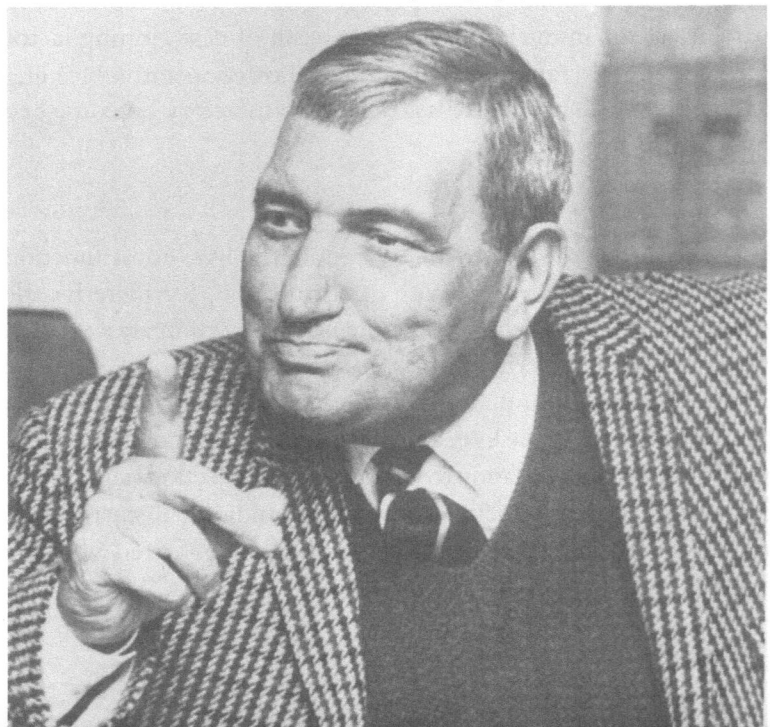

well from the start and the operation and post-operative course were, in each case, remarkably smooth and uncomplicated, upsetting the patients little more than any standard major surgical procedure. With the sound experimental background and some early clinical success there can be no doubt that liver grafting will in the future become established as satisfactory surgical treatment.

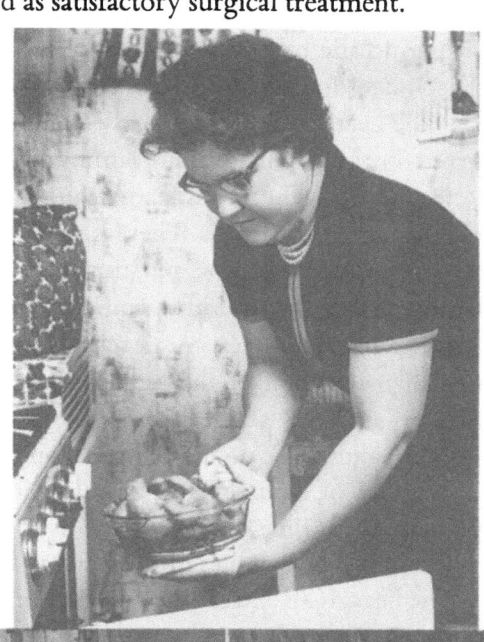

FIG. 36. Mrs. Winifred Smith one year after removal of her own diseased liver and transplantation of a liver from a dead donor. The severity of her liver disease would undoubtedly have killed her within a few weeks if she had not received a liver graft. She is now able to look after her family and live the life of a normal housewife.

ORGAN TRANSPLANTS

THE HEART

I doubt if there can be a mentally normal individual anywhere in the world who has not heard of heart transplantation and Professor Barnard, such is the efficiency of the mass media communication. A rather small minority of medical men, however, know that the technique of heart transplantation was developed over the preceding decade by Drs. Shumway, Lower, and their colleagues in the United States of America. It was these workers who showed that the heart could be regularly transplanted in dogs and would maintain the circulation until immunological rejection occurred. Rejection of the heart has features in no way distinguishable from rejection of other organs. There is a progressive cellular infiltration of the heart muscle and inflammatory changes in the coronary blood vessels, which lead to impairment of the circulation to the heart muscle itself. Heart graft rejection appears to be more aggressive than rejection of the kidney and more difficult to prevent. Nevertheless the standard immunosuppressive agents, Imuran, steroids, and ALG, do inhibit rejection for long periods in a small proportion of animals. The donor requirements for heart transplantation are the same as for the liver except that the heart will withstand a few minutes more of warm ischaemia time.

The heart is an extremely efficient pump with an inbuilt reliable power source and a regulatory mechanism providing versatility in performance, depending on the needs of the organism. At moments of fear and passion, the heart rate increases in speed and force so as to intrude on consciousness to an extent that can sometimes be alarming. Similar changes of function may occur in the bowels and ancient biblical scribes made reference to these bowel sensations in their theological texts. Prudish medieval translators substituted the word 'heart' for 'bowel'. Whether or not this was the source of the heart being the symbol of love and hate I do not know, but whatever the background there can be no doubt of the emotionally evocative nature of the word 'heart' and this, perhaps together with the long-established criterion of cessation of heartbeat as a sign of death, may explain the pathological interest that followed the first attempts at heart grafting in man. There are no differences in the objectives of heart transplantation to those of other organ grafts. If this simple fact was more widely appreciated, an explanation of organ transplantation would be greatly facilitated.

For some years surgeons have been able to treat defects of the heart valves and other cardiac abnormalities by direct surgery, with the heart stopped and its function temporarily taken over by an electrical pump. There are, however, certain disorders of the heart in which the heart muscle itself is permanently destroyed and replacement by a graft is the only conceivable treatment. For a heart graft to be of value it is essential that the patient is not suffering irreversible disease of other organs besides the heart. Coronary artery disease and certain degenerative conditions of heart muscle called 'cardiomyopathies' may lead to certain death solely by reason of disease localized to the heart. A patient suffering from such a fatal illness is a potential heart transplant recipient, since without a heart graft he will die. With the experimental background to which I have referred, a cautious approach to clinical heart grafting would seem to be fully justified. The first human heart graft was therefore a logical step forward, the surgery was well understood and the Cape Town team demonstrated clearly that the results of the animal investigations were applicable to man, and several patients have now survived more than a year after cardiac transplantation. It would have been preferable if clinical heart grafting had progressed in a similar manner to the development of kidney and liver grafting, namely in a few centres devoting much effort to the problem, with a well-established experimental background. Instead the immense prestige associated with the operation led to its performance all over the world by able cardiac surgeons, who often lacked any knowledge and even interest in transplantation immunology. When rejection resulted in the failure of many heart grafts it was not surprising that much bitter criticism resulted from those who had not benefited from the prestige and felt that the approach to heart transplantation had not been sufficiently serious. All organ transplantation suffered disastrously from this attack and instead of progress continuing it was abruptly halted. The evocative labels 'vulture' and 'vampire' were avidly seized by mass media and used in an irresponsible manner that is scarcely credible. The effect was a sudden loss of public confidence in the integrity of the medical profession and a suspicion that there could be a cynical disregard of human life in order to obtain organs for transplantation. These false and unfair judgements have interfered with organ transplantation programmes throughout the world by reducing the number of donors. In particular, many young patients with kidney disease, who could have been saved, are now dead—a very sad commentary on the way transplantation has been presented to the public.

THE LUNG

Techniques for grafting skin have been available for years and many people die from skin loss due to burns. A large percentage of these patients are young children who could be saved if only rejection of skin was preventable. It has already been explained that skin is probably the tissue most liable to rejection and immuno-suppressive methods that may keep kidney allografts functioning for years, delay rejection of skin grafts for only a few days or weeks. The reason for this is not known. Lung grafts can also be surgically transplanted with comparative ease and in animals autografts can function well indefinitely, but as with skin, it has been difficult to obtain good long-term results with lung allografts.

Lung function depends on exchange of gases between the air and the blood and the membrane across which the gases pass is an exceedingly delicate lining of the lung air spaces. Because of their necessary exposure to the air, lungs are more liable to infection than other organs, in fact pneumonia is one of the commonest causes of death after kidney, liver, or heart grafting. Infection of a grafted lung is therefore a particular hazard in patients given immuno-suppressive drugs. In addition the delicate air sac membrane is very easily damaged by a rejection reaction that would be mild and reversible in the kidney or liver, but once damaged gas exchange is seriously impaired and infection almost inevitable in the lung.

A complicated system of nerve connections between the lungs, brain, and chest muscles control breathing. If the nerves to and from both lungs are cut, breathing may be so unco-ordinated that death results. Transplantation of both lungs is therefore usually unsuccessful. Loss of one lung causes only moderate restriction of activity, therefore transplantation of one lung is a feasible proposition if the graft functions well.

Although chronic and eventually fatal lung disease is very common, by the time a patient is ill enough to consider lung trans-plantation, he is likely to be quite unfit for anaesthesia and opera-tion. With the rather poor results of experimental lung grafting and the other difficulties mentioned, it is not surprising that attempts at lung grafting in man have been few and unsuccessful. Infection has been the most common cause of death. The longest survivor was a Belgian patient who lived for six months. He was a young man with completely disabling fibrotic lung disease who received a lung graft from a cadaver. Initial function of the graft was excellent and the patient previously bedridden and continu-ously wedded to an oxygen mask, was able to leave hospital and return to activity. Rapid deterioration of lung function occurred shortly before death from a combination of rejection and infection.

The indications and scope of lung transplantation are unlikely to be defined until control of rejection is more effective and less toxic.

CHAPTER NINE

ETHICS AND THE LAW

To pour ridicule on and denigrate new ideas has been fashionable throughout history. It has usually taken years for life-saving advances to be accepted. Outstanding examples were Jenner's attempts to introduce vaccination against smallpox, Lister's advocacy of antiseptic surgery, and the early application of blood transfusion. The similar attitudes of some of the medical profession and public towards transplantation surgery is therefore not surprising; but we are now more used to rapid technical and scientific advances and change, so perhaps the phase of opposition may be short.

In Chapter Seven live donation of a kidney was discussed in relation to the age of the potential donor and his kinship to the recipient. The considerable difficulties that confront both the doctors and the family were explained and although kidney transplantation from live donors is often not possible or suitable, it was suggested that if there were no medical contra-indications and the potential donor, a close relative of the recipient, insisted that failure to proceed with the operation would result in a feeling of personal loss, then it was the duty of the doctors to perform the operation. The ethical situation with cadaver donors is surely much clearer. To be selected as an organ transplantation recipient means that no other treatment can save the patient's life and since a cadaver donor is dead, organ removal can do him no harm and its transplantation to the dying recipient may save his life. The need, objectives, and results of organ transplantation have been mentioned, why then is progress seriously impeded by shortage of donor organs when there could be more than sufficient suitable cadaver organs? Some of the reasons will be apparent to the reader, in particular the confused factual information available and certain emotional and irrational attitudes towards death, organ transplantation, and particularly the heart. In this chapter I will consider some of these matters in more detail.

DEATH AND RESUSCITATION

If a patient has a coronary thrombosis or is electrocuted or suffers from sudden brain injury or haemorrhage, there may be cessation of spontaneous respirations and/or effective heartbeat. Clearing the airway and performing artificial respiration is the time-honoured first aid treatment for such cases and is particularly well known in the context of drowning. If no resuscitative apparatus is available, mouth-to-mouth respiration can be effective; however, intubation of the trachea and mechanical ventilation of the lungs is more efficient and preferable. The heart may resume activity after ventilation has been restored and sometimes return of heartbeat appears to follow a sharp thump on the chest. If the heart fails to contract, artificial maintenance of the circulation by heart massage must be started within two to three minutes before irreversible brain damage occurs. Undoubtedly, many lives have been saved by these resuscitative methods, in particular, young patients with coronary thrombosis and those who have been electrocuted. It has, however, become customary practice to attempt resuscitation on every case of cardio-respiratory collapse. This would seem to be correct practice provided the patient is not known to be dying from an inevitably fatal disease, such as disseminated cancer so once commenced, when should resuscitation be abandoned? As far as the heart is concerned, attempts at cardiac massage should continue as long as there is evidence of electrical activity in the heart and there are signs of continuing brain function. Adequate cardiac massage should prevent dilatation of the pupils. Examination of the retina of the eye with an ophthalmoscope can be helpful. A normal appearance is an indication to continue resuscitation. Sludging and segmentation of blood in the retinal vessels are signs of death and together with intractably dilated pupils, and absent spontaneous cardio-respiratory activity, brain death is certain and attempts at resuscitation should be discontinued. To persist can do no good to the patient and will only distress the relatives. If, however, adequate circulation is restored but there is no spontaneous ventilation the question then arises as to how long mechanical ventilation should be continued. There are some who feel it should be continued until the circulation ceases, even if this may mean weeks, months, or even years of maintenance of the patient with obvious complete cerebral destruction—a tragic situation for those caring for a perfused but slowly decomposing corpse. The majority of medical men would regard this as bad medicine since it cannot possibly benefit the patient and will certainly cause anguish and distress to the relatives. Later they may even become indifferent, when they realize that the per-fused tissues they visit have no connection with the person they loved. Resuscitation should be continued whilst there is the slightest chance that the patient may recover; if, however, there is no evidence of central nervous activity, if the pupils are dilated and there is no electrical activity in the brain, then to persist with artificial ventila-tion is merely allowing the heart to perfuse a decerebrate corpse, analagous to keeping the decapitated body of a guillotine victim alive by artificial means. I have spent some time in discussion of this problem since it is, I hope, clear that the decision to stop resuscitation has absolutely nothing to do with any other consideration apart from the proper care of the patient himself. In particular, it has *nothing* to do with transplantation; but once the decision has been made, I believe it is the duty of the doctors concerned to inform the transplantation team and endeavour to obtain permission from the relatives of the dying person to remove organs for transplantation after death. After the mechanical ventilator has been turned off, removal of organs for transplantation does not commence until the circulation has ceased and death is obvious by traditional methods of diagnosis to any and every medical man and also to the nursing staff and laity.

When the circulation of blood ceases, death and putrefaction of the body follows. After three to five minutes at 37 °C the brain begins to suffer permanent damage and if the circulation is restored by artificial means, the brain damage will not allow the patient to recover, although the rest of the body cells may be alive. It is very important to realize the distinction between a live individual and living cells. Thus blood cells, cornea, or grafted organs can live after the death of the individual from whom they came and *per contra* an individual can live normally after removal of certain living tissues, such as the appendix or one kidney. A victim of the guillotine is dead following his decapitation—few people would question this—yet his heart may continue to beat for some minutes. In fact, if bleeding was controlled and the lungs ventilated with oxygen, all organs with the exception of the severed head could be kept alive for hours or even days, yet still no one would regard the individual as living. It follows that when destruction of the brain has been established, the individual has died no matter what the state of the rest of his body. This has led to the concept of 'brain death' or '*coma dépassé*' as a criterion of the individual's death, even though the heart continues to beat and provide a satisfactory circulation.

The diagnosis of brain death requires the following signs:

1. Deep, unrousable coma with fixed, dilated eye pupils, and absent cranial nerve reflexes.

2. No spontaneous respiration, the brain damage failing to provide the nervous control of respiration so that ventilation of the lungs must be maintained artificially by a machine.

3. Absence of electrical brain activity on the recording of an electro-encephalograph (EEG).

4. Cessation of circulation through the retina of the eye. This is a part of the brain that can be observed directly through the eye pupils with an ophthalmoscope.

5. Absent brain circulation determined by X-rays of the brain arteries after injection of radio-opaque material into them. In some cases these may be added the certain knowledge from operative exploration that the patient has a lethal brain injury or tumour.

If assessment of the above criteria is made by experienced doctors, there can be little chance of a mistake. In fact, as already explained, these are the usual indications to cease attempts at resuscitation, since persistence can do the patient no good and will only add to the relatives' distress in preserving a vegetable existence for a dead individual. Some doctors feel justified in removing organs for transplantation when 'brain death' has been diagnosed, before the heart has stopped beating. In fact, removal of the 'beating heart' for transplantation has been the routine policy in some centres in the United States. I am opposed to this practice and feel that it has led to much of the opposition to heart transplantation, since unless the brain has *been seen* to be removed, as in a guillotine victim, or is absent as in an anencephalic monster, there will always be the possibility that a mistake had been made, either due to human error or failure of the EEG machine. No matter how unlikely the chance of error, and I feel it is exceedingly unlikely, the fear is nevertheless present and would deter me from accepting the risk. Moreover, as has been seen, all organs can be successfully transplanted after traditional and unquestionable diagnosis of death following cessation of the circulation. Thus the criteria of brain death determines the need to cease attempts at resuscitation, for instance to withdraw mechanical lung ventilation. Cessation of the circulation will soon follow and death will then be quite certain. The lack of oxygen in the blood impairs the function of the heart so that effective heart contraction ceases and the circulation fails. After three to five minutes if there is no brain activity the brain must be dead and this means that the individual is dead. The ischaemic heart failure demonstrates beyond doubt that the previous assessment of brain death was correct. If a mistake had been made in assessing brain death the error would be revealed by resumption of spontaneous respiration by the patient with continued heartbeat and circulation.

I believe that this distinction is of great importance and is not just a technical quibble. Once the circulation has ceased in the presence of signs of brain death it is clear to any medical man, nurse, or indeed layman that the individual is dead and removal of organs for transplantation can do him no harm. To be of value the organs must be transplanted before they also die—organ removal and cooling must be quick. I believe it is quite justifiable at this stage after circulatory arrest to cool the whole body with a heart–lung perfusion machine and, if necessary, to restart the heart artificially if this facilitates transplantation. There can be no serious objection to this since the brain has been shown to be permanently dead.

Most deaths do not involve resuscitation and therefore the criteria required to cease resuscitation do not arise and death is diagnosed by cessation of the circulation and spontaneous respiration.

I hope the above discussion has clarified the often confused facts concerning resuscitation, 'turning off the machine', and diagnosis of death. In the very unusual situation where there may be difficulty in determining irreversible death, for example when the body is cold and circulation is maintained by an artificial heart–lung machine, the patient is considered to be alive until no doubts exist and brain death has been diagnosed. Only then is the heart–lung machine stopped and for reasons *totally* unrelated to transplantation considerations.

In most countries which have not introduced legislation specifically directed to the problem, the legal aspects of organ transplantation are ill defined. Laws relating to physical assault and care of the dead provide a legal framework quite unsuitable for organ transplantation. In the United Kingdom removal of an organ from a living person is technically an assault since the operation is not designed for that person's benefit. If, however, the safeguards referred to previously are adopted and the living donor has requested in writing that the operation be performed, then it is most unlikely that the doctors could be involved in court proceedings.

The Human Tissue Act of 1961 was introduced to facilitate corneal transplantation from cadavers. It was drafted before the need and feasibility of clinical organ transplantation were realized. A dead body is not property and therefore belongs to no one; it must, however, be treated with respect and not disfigured. The 1961 Act had certain ill-defined clauses which have never been tested in court. The principle that an individual's wishes as to the disposal of his own body should be respected was established, but no provision was made as to how these wishes relating to transplantation were to become available so that organ transplantation could be possible. If the deceased's wishes are not known then permission to remove organs for transplantation can be given by the relatives. If after 'undertaking such reasonable inquiry as may be practicable' the relatives cannot be contacted, then the person in charge of the body can give permission. Many deaths when the organs would be suitable for transplantation result from sudden accidents and, therefore, come under the jurisdiction of the coroner. He is responsible for investigating the cause of death and he can forbid organ removal.

If the deceased has on his body a card giving permission or forbidding removal of organs for transplantation then the situation is clear, but this is very unusual. Since preparations for organ removal must be made immediately after death it may be difficult or impossible to obtain permission in time, in which case the organs are wasted and potential recipients die. Yet often in these cases it transpires that the relatives explain too late that they would have given permission or that they knew it was the dead person's wish that his organs should have been transplanted. If the relatives can be contacted, to ask permission for organ removal can add to their distress. This is not always the case, even when the death of a young person has been sudden and unexpected. It is not unusual for the response to be 'I am glad you asked this, since I know it would have been his wish and at least some good may come from this terrible tragedy.' There are other cases, however, when the extreme misery of the bereaved relatives makes any discussion of organ removal an added pain that should be avoided. It may be difficult or impossible at the moment of terrible shock of bereavement, when a loved one, previously happy and healthy, has been killed in an accident, for the relatives to focus their minds on the question of organ removal. A day or so later it is much easier to discuss disposal of the body, but by then the organs are useless for grafting. One of the reasons for the shortage of donor organs is that fear of adding to the distress of the relatives by asking permission for organ removal causes the doctors who have cared for the dead patient to neglect the transplantation team by not informing them of the death.

There are some who feel that the supply of donor organs would be satisfactory if there was a widespread campaign encouraging people to volunteer to will their organs for transplantation after death, that is to 'contract-in'. This was the minority opinion of a committee set up to investigate this matter by the United Kingdom Government. I believe that most civilized people would prefer that their organs after death should help other human beings rather than be destroyed by cremation or devoured by worms. Nevertheless, I fear that it is most unlikely that there would be enough volunteers to be of practical value, since volunteering requires an active effort related to an unhappy thought, namely sudden unexpected death. The alternative proposal favoured by a majority of the committee was a 'contracting out' procedure, whereby permission to remove organs after death would be assumed unless specifically forbidden by the individual in his lifetime. This is the only way in which there can be enough organs to treat all those grievously in need of a transplantation. This proposal is not unprecedented. Legislation on these lines has already been accepted in Denmark, France, Sweden, Italy, and Israel. Moreover, compulsory post-mortem examination without any option of 'contracting-out' is routine practice after most sudden, unexpected deaths which come under the coroner's jurisdiction in the United Kingdom. A coroner's autopsy is a far more extensive procedure than organ removal for grafting, yet there has been no significant opposition to this sensible method of establishing the cause of death. I would regard the following safeguards as essential in a 'contracting-out' scheme.

1. The individual's wish should be the overriding consideration and it should be made easy for anyone to contract out on his own behalf and also on behalf of his children. He should be able to change his mind at any time and also specify which organs he does not want removed for transplantation, if he wishes to be selective. Since most people who would contract out feel strongly on the matter, I am sure they would register their objection immediately. The easiest way to object would be to fill in a prepaid card at a post office with one's name, age, and address. These details would be recorded on a central computer that could be contacted at any time of the day or night. As an additional safeguard, objectors could carry a card on their person stating their views. It would be helpful if those feeling strongly that they wanted their organs to be transplanted after death would register in a similar manner so that every effort would be made to comply with their wishes.

2. Diagnosis of death would follow the traditional, time-honoured observation of cessation of spontaneous respiration and circulation, following the principles outlined previously. Diagnosis of death should be made by doctors independent of the transplantation team. For cases on whom resuscitation had been attempted and abandoned, diagnosis of death should be the responsibility of two doctors, one of whom should have been qualified at least five years. *To be considered as a potential organ donor is the best safeguard against being sent to the mortuary whilst still alive, since death will be confirmed by a number of doctors and proof that there is no circulation will be established when, after an incision has been made to remove the organs, no bleeding results.*

3. If it was proposed to remove organs whilst the circulation continued, after *coma dépassé* had been diagnosed, permission of the relatives after full explanation would be necessary even in cases where the patient had 'contracted in' as a donor. In such cases signatures from two consultants experienced in neurology should testify to the brain death, and details would be given to the coroner.

4. The privacy of the bereaved relatives should not be abused by the press, radio, and television. The names, personal details, and photographs of donors and their relatives should not be made public even with the permission of those involved, since an effect of this publicity is to deter others from agreeing to be donors, for fear of being similarly treated. The coroner would safeguard the interests of the deceased and ensure that there had been no improper management in the terminal illness or organ removal.

5. There should be no changes in the care of the dying patient in order to facilitate organ transplantation. He should not be moved to another hospital unless he had specifically requested that this should be done for this purpose. In particular, unnecessary potentially dangerous investigations should not be performed. To remove

a small volume of blood for red cell grouping and tissue typing would be acceptable provided it did not upset the patient.

The only way in which there can be a sufficient supply of organs for transplantation is for legislation on the above lines to be adopted and for the public and medical profession to feel reassured that the transplantation doctors are following traditional medical ethical principles. This implies a bond of trust between the public and profession that is more important than any laws or safeguards. Trust between doctor and patient is fundamental in all medical care. When a surgeon advises a routine operation, the patient trusts him to have made a correct decision and to operate skilfully to the best of his ability. Exactly the same trust is involved in care of the dying, diagnosis of death, and organ removal. No matter what laws are passed, how many people are involved, or how numerous are the required criteria for establishing the diagnosis of death, in the end decisions are still made by human beings, who must be trusted to act according to accepted medical ethics. In my experience the mere thought of transplantation usually results in a renewal of efforts of the doctors and nurses in doing their utmost for the dying patient.

If a 'contracting out' scheme was accepted, although the law would not demand permission of the relatives, if the next of kin were available and could be approached without adding to their distress, they would always be consulted to confirm the wishes of the deceased, and if the relatives objected, even though the deceased had not, the doctors would respect their wishes, since to ignore them would be an act of inhumanity.

Most coroners are sympathetic to the needs of transplantation and will usually allow organ removal to proceed unless this would prevent them from establishing the cause of death. Organ removal is most unlikely to hinder the coroner's work. In fact, it may help him if the surgeon removing the organs reports any relevant finding to the coroner's pathologist. It is to be hoped that the small minority of unhelpful coroners will come to realize the unnecessary sadness they are causing to those dying of diseases that could be cured by organ grafts. Since the coroner is often unobtainable at the time of a death, a satisfactory procedure is for the transplantation doctors to confer with the coroner's pathologist. In this way the organ removal becomes the first stage of the coroner's post-mortem examination.

I have not so far considered the ethical aspects of recipient selection, except to point out that with the large number of young people dying from kidney disease without any offer of treatment, selection for kidney grafting must first be on medical grounds and then on a waiting-list basis. I am convinced that any method of assessing priorities on social grounds by 'independent, unbiased' panels can only lead to what will be regarded as invidious and prejudiced decisions, since opinions will differ widely on the impossible question as to 'what are the most worthy characteristics of citizenship?' The medical aspects of selection for an organ graft recipient are usually well defined and have already been considered. The prerequisite is fatal, untreatable disease of vital organs. No pressure is ever put on a patient to have an organ graft, in fact the reverse is true and many more patients request for and require organ transplantation than can be treated. It is the doctor's duty to be aware of the potential benefits of organ grafting for his patients and advise them and their relatives on the risks involved and the chances of success.

CHAPTER TEN

THE FUTURE

I have attempted to outline the background and present state of organ transplantation. In this chapter I will make some speculations on its future development. Forecasting is always a chancy business, particularly in such a fast-moving field as organ transplantation. Recent trends, however, have focused interest on certain aspects of the subject where knowledge is already sufficient to anticipate important advances in the foreseeable future. I will consider a few of these.

THE SURGERY

Surgical techniques are now available to transplant any organ. Refinements will undoubtedly make the various operative procedures safer and easier.

PREVENTION OF REJECTION

Although new drugs with less toxicity and more certain immuno-suppressive actions may be discovered, specific biological control of rejection by tolerance-inducing antigen is the ideal method of retaining a graft. Recent experimental findings concerning toler-ance induction in immunologically mature animals suggest that this goal may be attainable. If human histocompatibility antigens can be prepared in a form that would induce tolerance, there are two possible ways in which they might be used. It would be preferable to prepare the antigens from the organ donors so that it had just those specific determinants that were needed. It might, however, transpire that in order to produce tolerance, pretreatment with antigen would be necessary, in which case the organ donor's antigen could not be used but presumably antigen of identical specificity could be obtained from other sources. Thus one could envisage tissue typing a large number of cadavers, and preparing from them antigens of known specificity which could be stored and subsequently utilized to produce tolerance in recipients of organ grafts.

TISSUE TYPING

The principles of tissue matching have now been established and it is reasonable to predict with confidence that further development of current techniques will clarify tissue types to a similar extent to our present knowledge of red blood cell groups. It should then be feasible to assess with a high degree of accuracy the outcome of grafting between two matched individuals. Unfortunately, histocompatibility antigens are multiple and complicated, so that the chances of obtaining a perfect match will be small unless the pool of typed recipients and available donor organs is very large. Nevertheless the closer the match the better the chances of a successful graft and a good match means that graft rejection can be prevented with small safe doses of immunosuppressive agents. It is not impossible that the greatest value of tissue typing will eventually be its application to the production of specific immunological tolerance as explained above.

ORGAN PRESERVATION

It should soon be possible to preserve most organs with minimal deterioration for sufficient time for them to be transported many miles by air. Twelve to twenty-four hours of preservation may be achieved by relatively simple methods. I do not think, however, that it is likely that organ banks will be a reality in the foreseeable future. The idea of large numbers of organs being removed from tissue typed cadavers, their ischaemic damage repaired, and their safe preservation for weeks, months, or even years until required, is certainly attractive but will, I fear, remain a dream for some time to come.

LOGISTICS

To develop organ transplantation so as to utilize present knowledge will require extensive organization and co-operation. There are advantages in regional transplantation centres as opposed to individual hospitals transplanting different organs in small numbers. It is obviously economical and sensible to pool resources of tissue typing, organ preservation, immunosuppression, and dialysis. Doctors with specialized knowledge of these subjects would then be available to care for patients with grafts of different organs. Transplantation of any organ should be undertaken only by surgeons with training in vascular surgery. The more transplants performed by a given centre, the better the results are likely to be, due to the accumulated experience and continuous familiarity with the possible complications. This has been the case with other specialized surgical techniques.

For there to be sufficient organs to transplant, the law will need to be changed as suggested, and organs will need to be removed from patients that have died in all hospitals, not just in the transplantation centres. This will require close collaboration between doctors and hospitals so that the transplantation centre is informed of all suitable donors and surgeons trained in organ removal and preservation will be able to remove and conserve the organs before they are damaged, and arrange for their conveyance together with blood for tissue typing to the regional centre. It will be necessary for there to be a national organization in direct contact with the transplantation centres. The tissue types of all potential recipients would be registered at the national headquarters and when cadaver organs become available in a given centre the national organization would be notified and arrange for the dispatch of the organs to the nearest well-matched recipients. In certain cases it might be desirable to move the potential recipients to a transplantation centre some way off. I believe there is no indication to move a dying patient to a special hospital so that his organ can be more conveniently removed after death unless such a move was a specific wish of the dying man. It would then be justifiable to comply with the request provided the move was not prejudicial to his medical care. Such cases would be unusual.

If the national organization had no potential recipients of suitable tissue type then co-operation with the organizations of other countries should prevent organ wastage.

The above scheme is not the musing of idle speculation, such a system already exists in northern Europe, centred in Holland, under the direction of Professor J. J. Van Rood. This organization, Eurotransplant, already operates between the Benelux countries. There is a similar organization in Scandinavia. The requirements are computer facilities and an efficient twenty-four-hour transport service that may, when necessary, utilize aeroplanes or helicopters, although surface transport is more usual.

I often hear the view expressed that research effort in medicine devoted towards the care of the relatively few is unjustified when there are millions suffering from malnutrition or curable infectious diseases. It may well be that the human race will destroy itself by overpopulation exceeding all efforts at increased food production. The solution is clearly birth control within the limits of nutritional resources, but this straightforward concept becomes almost despairingly divorced from solution, when even a superficial consideration is given to human ignorance, superstition, and downright refusal to face facts in social organization and education. If the world population could be controlled then the benefits of modern preventive and therapeutic medicine would be available to all. These matters are, however, beyond the scope of my book and they are quite irrelevant as an argument against research into the treatment of relatively uncommon human disease. Pain and suffering are not confined to under-nourished, under-developed people. They occur with similar tragic features in the inhabitants of every country. Surely it is the duty and privilege of countries with a high standard of living to devote some of their financial resources to medical research into these diseases and their treatment. To neglect this opportunity would have a disastrous effect on intelligent medical inquiry and dampen the urge to discover new ideas and the workings of natural phenomena. Countries fortunate enough to be able to pursue medical research have an obligation to other less-fortunate countries to pursue this work. In due course the resulting advances will be applicable to all.

Another criticism of organ transplantation has been that research effort should instead be directed towards prevention of disease of vital organs. Certainly intense and continued effort should be made in disease prevention, but this need not and should not exclude work on organ transplantation. To work on a problem is no guarantee that it will be solved and important subjects such as the causes of cancer and atherosclerosis have not been discovered despite an immense expenditure of money and effort over many years. It may be necessary for new techniques and concepts at present quite unknown to be utilized in order to tackle these problem. Similar arguments apply to research into the causes and prevention of many of the fatal diseases of vital organs. On the contrary, I hope the discussions in this book have shown that the theoretical and developmental aspects of organ transplantation have sufficiently advanced to provide already life-saving treatment and progress continues to be so rapid that further important advances can be anticipated with reasonable confidence. This surely justifies continued and increased support for organ transplantation research.

The cost of a well-organized transplantation service is considerable, but in terms of alleviation of human suffering not excessive, and a mere drop in the ocean in relation to the defence budgets of most civilized countries. There are few who complain of the costs involved in the search for and rescue of shipwrecked sailors; planes and helicopters are used routinely. Why then should not a similar effort be made for those in an equally desperate plight with fatal disease involving a transplantable organ? The principles of a transplantation service are similar to those of a blood transfusion service and could be planned on comparable lines. The register of those 'contracting out' as donors could be linked to the national organization which would correlate tissue typing and organ transport. Commercial road, rail, and air transport would normally be used, but in emergencies at difficult times, such as public holidays and in the middle of the night, independent transport would need to be available. It is clear that the national organization would have to be staffed by highly trained individuals with considerable specialized knowledge.

I hope this short book has explained and clarified some aspects of organ transplantation. In the future increasing numbers of vital organs will be transplanted successfully and, accordingly, become less and less newsworthy. If safe immunosuppression is developed, other organs, such as the pancreas, intestines, and even skin, will be transplanted in preference to less-satisfactory conventional treatment. For this development to proceed it will be necessary for the public and medical profession to view cadaver organ removal as the routine procedure in suitable cases. It will become apparent that a doctor's failure to notify the regional transplantation team of a potential donor is unethical medical conduct, since patients awaiting grafting will die unnecessarily as a consequence. It may one day be possible to transplant organs from animals to man with success, but this is unlikely to be achieved until grafts from man to man are uniformly successful. In the meantime in a welfare state, where all are supposed to have equal opportunity for medical treatment, we should consider with more compassion the many young people who are being allowed to die due to shortage of organs for transplantation.

Most of us would make every endeavour to save a man drowning, many would risk life and limb in the attempt. To donate one's organs after death is a similar act of charity that involves no risk at all yet can provide another human being with a gift of life.

GLOSSARY

Adhesions. Abnormal sticking together of organs in the abdominal cavity, usually developing after an operation on the abdomen.

Adenine. An important constituent of the nucleic acids.

Adrenal cortex. The outer core of the adrenal glands which are paired organs, one lying on top of each kidney. They produce steroids which are important in regulating the salt and water balance of the body.

Agglutination. The clumping together of cells which are normally freely suspended in a fluid, for example, blood. Agglutination often occurs in the presence of antibodies which can react with the antigens on the surfaces of the cells.

Albumin. A protein, similar to egg white, which is found in the blood.

Allergic reaction. An immune response to a foreign material which results in damage to the body's own tissues. For example, pollen acts as an antigen and the response to it causes the familiar symptoms of hay fever.

Allograft. A graft taken from one individual of a species and transplanted into another individual of the same species.

Anastomosis. Surgical junction of hollow structures e.g. joining together a severed artery to restore blood flow through it.

ALG. See anti-lymphocyte globulin.

ALS. See anti-lymphocyte serum.

Amino acids. The nitrogen-containing substances which are the building blocks of which proteins are made.

Anencephalic monster. Child born without a brain.

Antibodies. When any foreign material gains entry to the body, it is recognized as foreign by the lymphoid system. Within seven to ten days the lymphoid system manufactures proteins called antibodies. Foreign materials which stimulate the formation of antibodies in this way are known as antigens. The antibodies, when they are formed, combine with the antigens. If the antigens are free poisonous substances, the combination with antibodies may inactivate them and abolish their toxicity. If the antigens are attached to cells, such as bacteria or red blood cells, the cells may be destroyed by combination with the antibody. When the same individual is exposed to a particular antigen a second time, the lymphoid system is capable of recognizing that it has met with the antigen previously. It then produces large amounts of antibody very quickly. It is important to realize that each antibody is specific to a particular antigen; an antibody which has been manufactured in response to one foreign protein will not usually react with a different type of foreign protein.

—, **blocking.** Antibodies which react with the antigens on the cells of a transplanted organ without destroying those cells. The antigens are thus covered up and no longer provoke an immune response. Blocking antibodies may thus protect an organ against rejection the process is called 'enhancement' since the continued survival of the graft is enhanced.

—, **cytotoxic.** Antibodies capable of killing cells and tissues.

—, **enhancing.** See antibodies, blocking.

Anticoagulation. Reduction of the clotting activity of the blood, usually by means of drugs.

Antigens. Substances which, when they gain entry to the body, are capable of provoking an immune response. Part of this response involves the manufacture of antibodies. Another part involves the action of the cells of the lymphoid system on the foreign material. Antigens may be free chemical substances or, more important in the case of blood transfusions and organ transplants, attached to cell membranes.

—, **histocompatibility.** Antigens attached to cells which enable one individual to recognize the cells of another individual as foreign. Red blood cells carry two important antigens, A and B. If the red cells of two individuals carry the same antigens then blood can be transfused from one to another without disaster. Similar antigens on other body cells that lead to rejection after transplantation are called 'histocompatibility antigens'.

GLOSSARY

Anti-lymphocyte globulin, ALG. If serum proteins· are analysed one component is called globulin and this contains most of the antibodies. The globulin from anti-lymphocyte serum is called anti-lymphocyte globulin.

Anti-lymphocyte serum, ALS. When lymphocytes of one species are injected into an animal of another species, the recipient produces a whole range of antibodies against antigens carried on the surfaces of the injected lymphocytes. If blood from the recipient is collected and the red and white cells are removed, the resulting clear, straw-coloured fluid containing the antibodies is known as anti-lymphocyte serum. When this serum is injected into an individual of a species from which the original lymphocytes came, it will destroy the lymphocytes in that individual. Unfortunately, some of the antigens on the lymphocytes are also found on red cells and the serum as well as destroying lymphocytes may destroy red cells and provoke dangerous reactions. The serum must, therefore, be modified by incubating it with an excess of red cells *in vitro* before injection. These react with and remove the antibodies which destroy red cells leaving only the antibodies which destroy lymphocytes specifically.

Aorta. The main blood vessel carrying blood from the heart.

Arterio-venous fistula. An artificial connection made directly between an artery and a vein.

Autograft. A graft taken from one part of an individual and put in another part of the same individual. Skin grafts used in plastic surgery are examples.

Artery. A blood vessel carrying fresh, oxygenated blood away from the heart to the tissues of the body.

—, renal. The artery to the kidney.

Auto-immune disease. Disease caused by the immune mechanism of an individual turning against one or more of its own organs.

Azathioprine. The proper chemical name of Imuran, an important immunosuppressive drug.

Bacteria. Single-celled organisms found virtually everywhere in the environment as well as on the skin and in the gut. Most bacteria are harmless to man, some are even useful; others, called pathogenic bacteria, may cause disease on gaining entry to the body.

Bile. The secretion produced by the liver. It is stored in the gall bladder and flows down the bile duct into the duodenum. It is important in the digestion of fats and contains some waste matter.

Biliary cirrhosis. A disease of the liver which follows blocking or congenital absence of the bile ducts.

Blocking antibodies. See antibodies, blocking.

Blood groups. Like other cells the red cells of the blood have antigens on their surfaces. The red cells can be destroyed if they come into contact with antibodies to these antigens. Only three antigens are of major importance, A, B, and Rh. It is, therefore, relatively simple to determine an individual's blood group by examining his red cells to see which of these antigens they carry. Blood from an individual of one group given to another individual of the same group will provoke no reaction and will be safe.

Bone marrow. The cavity found in the centre of many bones is filled with the soft tissue known as bone marrow. The marrow manufactures both red and white blood cells. It is very susceptible to damage by radiation.

Bronchus. The airway leading from the trachea to the lungs.

Cadaver. Corpse.

Cell. All organs are made up of myriads of tiny sub-units known as cells. The very simplest animals and plants may consist of only a single cell, for example a bacterium.

—, endothelial. The delicate cells lining blood vessels.

—, mononuclear. White cells in the blood having a single rounded nucleus. Most of them belong to the lymphoid system.

—, plasma. Cells formed from lymphoid tissue which manufacture antibodies.

—, red blood. The cells which are freely suspended in blood and which because they contain the pigment haemoglobin make the blood red. They are vital for the transport of oxygen around the body.

Cirrhosis. A disease in which the normal cells of the liver are damaged and replaced by fibrous tissue which tends to grow in a disordered and excessive manner. It may be caused by over-indulgence in alcohol, by blockage of the bile ducts, or by hepatitis, but in many cases the cause is unknown.

GLOSSARY

Clotting factors. Clotting of the blood requires more than a dozen different substances. These are known as the clotting factors and most of them are manufactured by the liver.

Colitis. Inflammation of the large bowel (colon).

Coma dépassé. Total and inreversable brain death with the heart still beating and the lung being ventilated mechanically.

Cornea. The transparent part of the front of the eyeball.

Coronary thrombosis. Blocking of one of the arteries to the heart leading to a 'heart attack'.

Cortex, adrenal. See adrenal cortex.

Cortisone. A synthetic substance which has some of the actions of the natural adrenal steroid hormones.

Cranail nerves. The twelve paired nerves that are connected directly to the brain.

Cushing's syndrome. A disease caused by an excess of adrenal cortical hormones in the body.

Cytotoxicity. Ability to destroy cells.

Cytoxic antibodies. See antibodies, cytotoxic.

Deletion of histocompatibility antigens. When a transplant has been in an individual for some time there may be a loss of antigens from the surfaces of the transplant cells. This may enable the dose of immunosuppressive drugs to be reduced without rejection occurring. See antibodies, blocking.

Diabetes mellitus. A disease in which the pancreas fails to produce enough of the hormone insulin. Insulin is vital for the handling of carbohydrates such as sugar and starch.

Dialysis. The removal from the blood of harmful waste products and water which may accumulate in excess when the kidneys fail. In the form known as haemodialysis the blood is taken out of the body, put through a machine where it is purified, and then returned to the body.

Electro-encephalography. The recording of the electrical activity of the brain via electrodes placed on the skull.

Endothelial cells. See cells, endothelial.

Enhancing antibodies, enhancement. See antibodies, blocking.

Enzymes. Protein substances in the body which are essential for certain chemical reactions which occur. Each reaction usually has its own special enzyme.

Fibrin. A protein found in the blood which forms the meshwork of a blood clot.

Follicles, lymphoid. Aggregations of lymphoid cells.

Fractionation. Separation into basic components, for example, breaking cells down into cell membrane nuclei, cytoplasm, etc.

Fundus, optic. The back of the inside of the eyeball which can be seen through the pupil using an instrument known as an ophthalmoscope.

Gastritis. Inflammation of the stomach.

Glomerulonephritis. A disease of the kidneys which may follow a throat infection by an organism known as the streptococcus. Unfortunately antigens carried by certain streptococci seem in some people to be similar to the antigens carried by their own kidneys. Parts of the kidneys may, therefore, be accidentally destroyed during the immune response to the streptococcus.

Glycoprotein. A complex substance containing both carbohydrate and protein.

Graft, homo-. A graft from one individual of a species to another individual of the same species—i.e. a synonym of allograft.

—, allo-. See allograft.

—, auto-. See autograft.

—, orthotopic. A graft put in the place in the body where the organ which the graft is replacing is normally found.

—, heterotopic. A graft put in an unusual place in the body.

—, second-set. A homograft does not usually begin to be rejected until seven to ten days after transplantation as it takes that time for the recipient to mount an immune response when it meets with new antigens for the first time. But with a second graft from the same donor, rejection begins virtually immediately. This is known as the second-set phenomenon.

Graft *v*. host reaction. If lymphoid tissue or lymphocytes from another individual are put into a host whose immune response is defective (e.g. because of treatment with immunosuppressive agents), the donor cells may destroy the tissues of the recipient (host) instead of the other way round.

Haemodialysis. See dialysis.

Hepatectomy. Removal of the liver.

Hepatitis. Inflamation of the liver usually due to a virus infection.

Heterotopic grafts. See graft, heterotopic.

Histocompatibility factors. See antigens, histocompatibility, and also deletion of histocompatibility antigens.

Homograft. See graft, homo-.

Immune response. The response of the body to any foreign material gaining access to the body. See also antigen, antibodies, lymphoid tissue, and allergic reaction.

Immunization. The exposure of the body to a particular antigen or set of antigens resulting in a much quicker response to a second exposure to the same antigens. This is important in resisting infections and explains why some diseases such as chicken pox or measles are caught only once; the disease is nipped in the bud after the first time. With many diseases such as poliomyelitis and smallpox, vaccines are available which carry all the antigens of the virulent disease-causing organisms yet which do not cause the disease themselves. The body thus responds quickly on exposure to the real organism and the disease does not develop. Immunization is also important in allergic responses and in the second-set phenomenon.

Immunoblasts. A type of lymphoid cell important in the immune response.

Immunological tolerance. A situation in which an individual does not mount a response against a foreign antigen. Exposure to foreign antigens in foetal life induces immunological tolerance to those antigens if encountered subsequently.

Immunosuppressive drugs. Drugs which inhibit the immune response, so reducing the risk of rejection of a transplanted organ. Unfortunately at the same time the risk of infection is greatly increased.

Inbreeding. The close breeding of related individuals which after many generations may mean that all the individuals concerned have a similar genetic constitution and can thus accept transplants from one another.

Intubation. Insertion of a tube into the windpipe in order to connect the lungs to an artificial respiration machine.

Insulin. A hormone produced by the pancreas which is deficient in diabetes mellitus.

In utero. In the womb.

In vivo. In the living body.

In vitro. Literally in glassware, outside the living body in the laboratory.

Ischaemia. Absence of an adequate blood supply to an organ.

—, warm ischaemia time. The interval after death before the organ to be transplanted can be cooled. Ideally this period should be as short as possible.

Kidneys. A pair of organs lying in the abdominal cavity which are responsible for controlling the output of unwanted water, salt, and waste material in the urine.

Liver. The major chemical factory in the body. It is a single organ lying high up in the abdominal cavity. It is largely responsible for the processing of digested food which it receives from the gut via the portal vein, for the detoxification of many poisons, for the storage of important substances like vitamin A, and for the manufacture of the proteins and clotting factors of the blood.

Lungs. The organs via which oxygen is taken into the blood and the waste product, carbon dioxide, leaves it.

Lymph. In the tissues some fluid escapes from the blood. This is lymph, and it is collected by a system of tubes known as the lymphatics and eventually emptied back into a vein. The tissues from which lymph comes may contain abnormal material such as dirt, bacteria, or cancerous cells. The lymph passes through collections of lymphoid tissue known as lymph nodes where the lymph is filtered and the abnormal material is prevented from reaching the blood.

Lymphoid tissues. All the tissues in the body concerned with the lymphatic system. They include the lymph nodes, spleen, thymus, bone marrow, tonsils, and appendix.

Lymphoid follicles. See follicles, lymphoid.

GLOSSARY

Lymphocytes. Small white cells found in the blood and lymphatic system. They are manufactured in the lymphoid tissue and are essential for the immune response.

Metabolism. A general word used to cover all the chemical reactions which go on in the body.

Metabolites. Products of metabolism.

Monozygotic twins. See twins, monozygotic.

Marrow bone. See bone marrow.

Mononuclear cells. See cells, mononuclear.

6-mercaptopurine. An anti-leukaemic drug from which the immuno-suppressive drug Imuran was derived.

Nephrectomy. Removal of a kidney.

Nervous reflex. Unconcious muscular response to a stimulus, e.g. blinking of the eyelid when the eyeball is touched.

Neuritis. Damage to peripheral nerves leading to defects of sensation and muscle function.

Oedema. The accumulation of fluid outside the blood vessels and in the tissues. Its old name is dropsy. It is particularly common around the ankles in heart failure and kidney disease.

Ophthalmoscope. See fundus, optic.

Optic fundus. See fundus, optic.

Orthotopic graft. See graft, orthotopic.

Pancreas. An important organ in the abdomen. It produces the pancreatic juice which is essential for digestion and also manufactures insulin.

Perfusate. Fluid used to perfuse an organ.

Pericarditis. Inflammation of the pericardium (the fibrous membrane covering the heart).

Plasma cells. See cells, plasma.

Platelets. Tiny fragments of cells found in the blood which are essential for the normal clotting of blood.

Pneumonia. Infection of the lung tissues.

Polycystic disease. An inherited disease of the kidneys. Many cysts are formed in the organs and eventually the kidneys are destroyed.

GLOSSARY

Portal vein. See vein, portal.

Prednisone and Prednisolone. Synthetic drugs which have many of the actions of the adrenal cortical hormones.

Prosthesis. An artificial replacement for an organ, for example, an artificial limb or plastic heart valves.

Radio-opaque material. Material which is impervious to X-rays and, therefore, causes a shadow on an X-ray picture. Such material may be used to show up the stomach (barium meal) or when injected into the blood to outline the course of a vessel.

Rejection. The destruction by the body's immune response of an organ or tissue transplanted from another individual.

Renin. A substance produced by damaged or ischaemic kidneys which leads to a raised blood pressure.

Scribner shunt. A plastic tube making a connection between an artery and vein which can be used to connect a patient to a dialysis machine.

Second-set phenomenon. See graft, second-set, and also immunization.

Serological tissue typing. The process by which the antigens carried by a person are identified.

Serum. The clear fluid left when a blood clot is formed. It contains most of the proteins found in the blood apart from the clotting factors which are used up in the clot.

Shock. A state of persistent low blood pressure which may follow haemorrhage, extensive burning, or a number of other abnormal events.

Shunt, Scribner. See Scribner shunt.

Steroids. See adrenal cortex.

Thrombocytopaenia. A deficiency of platelets in the blood often leading to defective clotting.

Thrombosis. Abnormal clotting of the blood inside blood vessels.

Thymectomy. Removal of the thymus.

Thymus. A gland found inside the chest which is essential for the normal development of the lymphoid system.

Thyroid. A gland found at the front of the neck. It produces thyroid hormone which is essential for the control of all the chemical reaction in the body.

GLOSSARY

Tissue matching. The process by which the antigens found on a potential organ donor's cells are matched as closely as possible with those on the cells of a potential recipient.

Tolerance. See immunological tolerance.

Trachea. The windpipe.

Twins. There are two types of twins. In one case (identical or mono-zygotic) only one egg fuses with one sperm to give a single fertilized egg. Both twins come from this single egg and, therefore, they have identical genetic composition. In the other case (non-identical or dizygotic) two sperms fuse with two eggs. The twins are genetically quite distinct and are no more likely to resemble one another very closely than are ordinary brothers and sisters.

Uraemia. The term given to the condition of the patient in terminal renal failure. The blood levels of the waste product urea are very high but this is not the cause of all the unpleasant symptoms.

Vein. A blood vessel returning deoxygenated blood from the tissues to the heart and lungs.

Virus. An organism smaller than bacteria which can only live as a parasite in the cells of another individual. Many important diseases such as smallpox and poliomyelitis are caused by viruses.

LIST OF PERSONS
MENTIONED IN THE TEXT

BARNARD, C. N. Professor of cardiovascular surgery, Cape Town.

BRESCIA, M. J. Physician at the Renal Service Dialysis Unit, Veterans Administration Hospital, Bronx, New York.

BURNET, Sir Macfarlane. Former Director of the Walter and Eliza Hall Memorial Institute, Melbourne, Australia. Nobel Prize 1960 (Medicine).

CARREL, Alexis, 1873–1944. French experimental surgeon and biologist. Nobel Prize, 1912 (Physiology and Medicine), for work in developing a new method for suturing blood vessels.

CIMINO, J. E. Chief, Renal Service Dialysis Unit, Veterans Administration Hospital, Bronx, New York.

DAVIES, D. A. L. Biochemist and immunologist. Searle Research Laboratories, High Wycombe.

GOWANS, J. Royal Society Professor and Director, Medical Research Council Cellular Immunology Research Unit, Oxford.

LOWER, Richard E. Professor of cardiovascular surgery, Richmond, Virginia.

MEDAWAR, Sir Peter. British biologist. Director of National Institute for Medical Research. Nobel Prize, 1960 (Physiology and Medicine).

METCHNIKOFF, E. 1845–1916. Russian biologist. Nobel Prize (jointly with Paul Ehrlich), 1908 (Medicine), for work in immunity. Chief work, while in Paris, on immunity of infectious diseases.

MILLER, J. A. F. P. Immunologist. Walter and Eliza Hall Memorial Institute, Melbourne, Australia.

MOORE, Francis D. Moseley Professor of Surgery, Harvard Medical School. Surgeon-in-Chief, Peter Bent Brigham Hospital, Boston.

PERSONS MENTIONED IN THE TEXT

MURRAY, Joseph E. American plastic surgeon at Peter Bent Brigham Hospital, Boston. Assistant Professor of Surgery, Harvard Medical School.

SCRIBNER, B. Nephrologist, Seattle.

SHUMWAY, Norman E. Professor of cardiovascular surgery, Stanford University, Palo Alto, California.

STARZL, Thomas E. Professor of surgery, Denver, Colorado.

VAN ROOD, J. J. Professor of immunology, Leiden, Netherlands.

WOODRUFF, Sir Michael. Professor of Surgical Science, University of Edinburgh, and surgeon, Edinburgh Royal Infirmary.

INDEX

INDEX

INDEX

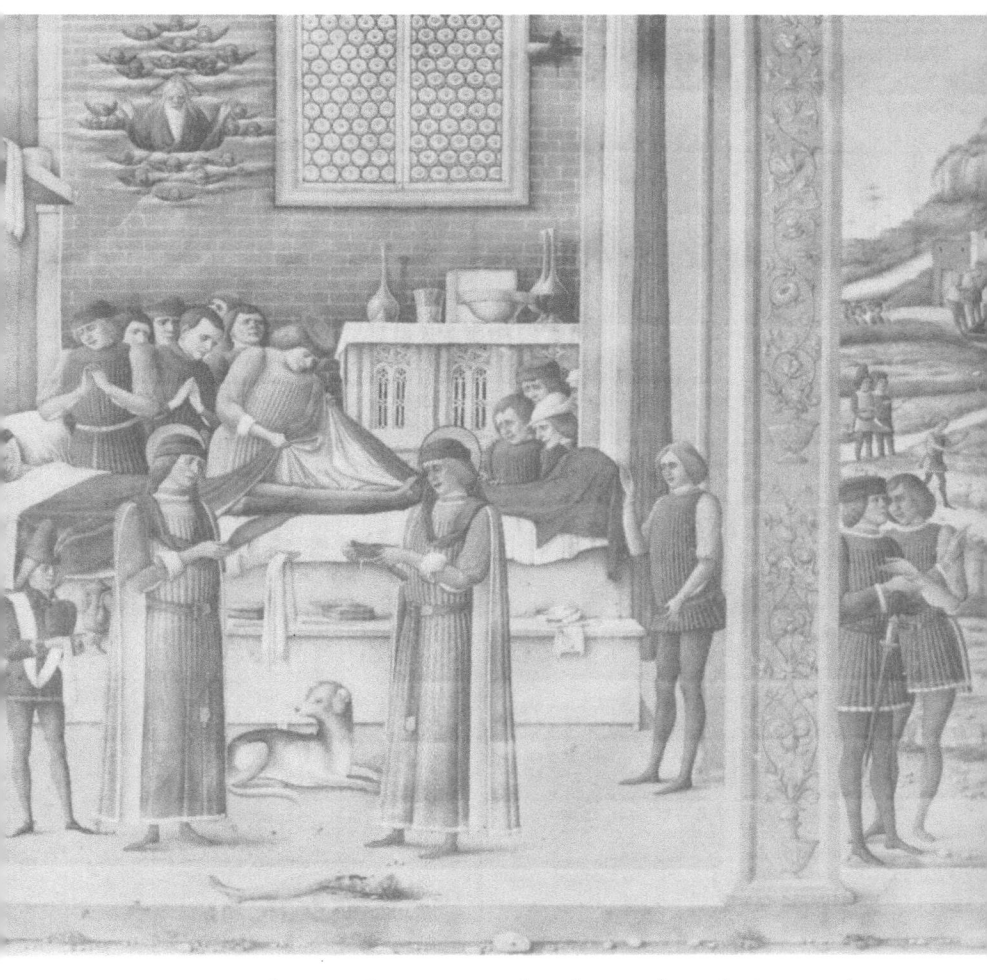

FIG. 1. Reproduction of a painting attributed to Girolamo da Cremona (1463–5) of Saints Cosmas and Damian transplanting a leg from a dead donor to a patient afflicted with a tumour of his leg (appearing in 'Brooke Antiphonal', Society of Antiquaries).